AN OVERVIEW OF PSYCHIATRIC MEDICATION

2nd Edition

Christian Jonathan Haverkampf MD

PPC
Psychiatry Psychotherapy Communication
Publishing Ltd

An Overview of Psychiatric Medication

Psychiatry Psychotherapy Communication
Publishing Ltd

Published by Psychiatry Psychotherapy Communication
Publishing Ltd
Dublin

First published in the United States of America by
Psychiatry Psychotherapy Communication
Publishing Ltd
San Francisco, CA, USA

Copyright © 2017-2018 Christian Jonathan Haverkampf
All rights reserved.
Unauthorized reproduction and/or publication in any form is prohibited.

Printed in the United States of America
Set in Calibri

Except in the United States of America, this book is sold subject to the condition that it shall not, by way of trade or otherwise, be lent, resold, hired out, or otherwise circulated without the publisher's prior consent in any form of binding or cover other than that in which it is sold and without a similar condition including this condition being imposed on the subsequent purchaser.

The scanning, uploading and distribution of this book via the Internet or via any other means without the permission of the publisher is illegal and punishable by law. Please purchase only authorized electronic editions, and do not participate in or encourage electronic piracy of copyrighted materials. Your support of the author's rights is appreciated.

Table of Contents

Introduction ... 1

Depression ... 3

Anxiety, Panic Attacks ... 13

Obsessive Compulsive Disorder (OCD) ... 26

Insomnia ... 39

Bipolar Disorder ... 50

Social Anxiety ... 66

Schizophrenia ... 71

Trauma ... 77

Attention Deficit Hyperactivity Disorder (ADHD) ... 80

Tourette's ... 93

Weight Gain and the Metabolic Syndrome ... 95

Psychiatric Emergencies ... 105

QT Prolongation ... 118

Serotonin Syndrome ... 139

The Combination with Psychotherapy ... 151

Suicide Prevention ... 155

Monitoring for Antidepressants ... 168

Monitoring for Antipsychotics ... 179

IMPORTANT NOTICE & DISCLAIMER

The publisher and author cannot assume any responsibility or liability for any injuries or losses including any present and/or future physical or psychological pain or injury that anyone incurs, as a result of acting upon any information provided by this book.

This book is solely a basis for academic discussion among medical professionals and no medical advice is given. The information contained herein may be false, inaccurate, omitting important information and/or outdated. The lists of drugs have not been checked for accuracy or completeness. Consult a professional if you believe you might suffer from a medical condition.

Trademarks belong to their respective owners. Even if a word is not marked as such, it may still be trademarked. No checks have been made to this effect.

Introduction

Psychiatric medication is used to treat mental illnesses. Usually prescribed in psychiatric settings, these medications are typically made of synthetic chemical compounds. Mostly they influence the neurotransmitter makeup in the vast network of nerve cells (neurons) that make up the brain.

Medication and psychotherapy are not mutually exclusive. Psychiatric Medication can also be used as a short- and medium-term support to a long-term focused psychotherapy. Most common psychotherapeutic approaches are compatible with the use of medication, such as cognitive behavioral therapy (CBT), psychodynamic psychotherapy, interpersonal therapy (IPT) and communication-focused therapy, which was developed by the author.

Psychiatric drugs have helped treat conditions in outpatient settings, that often required lifelong hospitalization in the centuries before. They are also effective in the treatment of anxieties, depression, panic attacks and many conditions that may also be to a significant degree a result of the environment we all live in and a lack of adequate psychological strategies to deal with it, while pursing one's values, interests and aspirations.

All medication can have side-effects

No medication is potentially without side-effects. Some psychiatric medications can also lead to interactions with each other or with non-psychiatric drugs. However, many psychiatric drugs are quite safe as compared to other non-psychiatric medication. One reason may be that it is much more difficult to get registration for psychiatric medication than for medication to treat severe medical conditions, even if both have roughly the same side-effects. People generally expect medication to treat moderate mental health conditions to be as close to "safe" as possible.

Another reason for a high standard of safety is that the occurrence of adverse effects can potentially reduce drug compliance much more in drugs used to treat mental health conditions. Some adverse effects can be treated symptomatically by using adjunct medications such as anticholinergics (antimuscarinics). Some rebound or withdrawal adverse effects, such as the possibility of a sudden or severe emergence or re-emergence of psychosis in antipsychotic withdrawal, may appear when the drugs are discontinued, or discontinued too rapidly. [A]

Depression

The Faces of Depression

Depression comes in a multitude of flavors. Traditionally a distinction has been made between the reactive or neurotic depression on one end, which has been seen largely as environmentally induced, and the endogenic depression, which was largely seen as driven by the patient's biology. We now know that all three factors of biology, psychology and environment interact together in the pathogenesis of depression. However, when it comes to medication, the distinction between largely environmentally induced depressions and those where no triggering event is apparent, the largely biological one, can be important. In cases of reactive depressions, for example in the context of burnout or very stressful life situations, medication may not work as fully and as quickly as it does in the depressions 'out of the blue' with a more strongly biological 'feel'.

The Circularity of Depression

Due to the plasticity of the brain, which regulates its morphological and chemical balance all the time, environmental influences can affect the circuitry and the functioning of the brain. Since the biology of the brain determines our thoughts and actions, it influences our environment, which again has a feedback on the brain. Thus, all effect depends on communication inside the brain and between the brain and the environment, and vice versa. This plays an immense role in the etiology and the symptoms of depression. It also explains why a combination of medication and psychotherapy in the majority of cases has the best outcome. Medication should be thought of in many cases of depression, except for the lighter reactive versions, while psychotherapy is always indicated if an individual suffers from depression. A condition that relies largely on communication deficits to be maintained, can also be cured through the 'talking cure', psychotherapy.

The Combination of Psychotherapy and Medication

Depression should in any case be treated with a combination of psychotherapy and medication if it is serious enough. Psychotherapy in most cases takes a few months to work, and medication, while also requiring a few weeks to work, will in many cases get results quicker than psychotherapy alone. In less severe cases, especially when it is a reaction to obvious external factors, psychotherapy alone may do. Medication can especially provide relief before the effect of psychotherapy, which is more geared towards the long-run, takes hold. While medication cannot make life more meaningful per se, it can improve an individual's mood, which usually leads to more positive thoughts, a more positive outlook on the world, a decrease in ruminations, less anxiety and improved sleep – and appetite if that is desired.

Suicidal Ideation

Suicidality needs to be kept in mind in any form of depression and the mainstream opinion has shifted towards addressing these thoughts rather than avoiding talking about them out of fear that it might trigger them. Since the stability of the therapeutic relationship and communication itself are important tools in relieving depression, one should not be too anxious about naming issues that seem relevant.

A concern was that since the activating effect in several antidepressants can occur before the antidepressant affect, the risk for suicide might increase because a patient who still feels depressed becomes more active. However, the clinical experience is that the opportunity to talk about feelings and thoughts openly in a secure relationship reduces the urge towards self-harm.

Interests and Values

As I have outlined in another article on depression, facilitating the vision of a future the patient has some control over is often an important step in treating depression. This often means identifying values, interests and aspirations, which can provide greater motivation and a good feeling about the future, should be allowed enough space. There can be sadness about lost opportunities, but this usually subsides in the face of having a clearer direction in life and a greater promise of happiness, if one pursues the things one truly values and aspires to.

Medication

Unfortunately, the perfect medication does not exist. But this is also not to be expected since each antidepressant has a unique profile of effects, positive and negative, which can still be influenced largely by the unique biology of the patient. The following antidepressants are the most common ones. Using a single antidepressant (monotherapy) is usually to be preferred over polypharmacy. However, especially in more severe and treatment-resistant cases of depression, combinations may have to be explored, such as combining venlafaxine and mirtazapine ("California rocket fuel") to yield an especially potent antidepressant and activating combination, which can even improve sleep (at lower to medium doses of mirtazapine).

Selective serotonin reuptake inhibitors (SSRIs)

The selective serotonin reuptake inhibitors (SSRIs) are the most common used antidepressants because of their relative safety and low side-effect profile. Unfortunately, in the beginning the indiscriminate use of the SSRI Prozac® against 'everything' from workplace problems to the stress of unhealthy living lead to a backlash in the media, which unfortunately made many patients avoid all medication out of fear to become emotionally flat or experience a change in one's personality, which has not been shown so far in any convincing way.

There are several other substances, that work as antidepressants, and all have potential side-effects. Often a substance is used which has a 'desirable' side-effect and that deals more effectively with the individual constellation of symptoms:

Insomnia

Mirtazapine (Remeron® and many generics) is effective in inducing sleep at lower doses (around 15mg), an effect that seems to wear off once one goes up to 45mg. However, the antidepressant effect of 15mg is usually too small. Especially early on 'hangovers' in the morning are not uncommon. Among very common side effects are dry mouth, constipation, increased appetite, as well as somnolence, sedation, sleepiness (which may wear off).

Initiative, Motivation

Lack of activation: Venlafaxine (Effexor®, Effexor XR®, Lanvexin®, Viepax®, Trevilor®) is a noradrenaline and serotonin reuptake inhibitor (NSRI) and often affectively increases activation. However, one should be careful with patients who might harm themselves (or others) because activation often occurs before the antidepressant effect takes hold. Also, if used in cases of anxiety it may increase the anxiety before reducing it.

Anxiety, Panic Attacks, OCD

Co-morbidity with anxiety, panic attacks, OCD: the SSRIs are a good first choice. Venlafaxine seems to be helpful with anxiety, but often it increases anxiety early on, and possibly even medium-term.

Tricyclic antidepressants

Tricyclic antidepressants should not be used to treat symptoms that can be treated with the SSRIs or an NSRI, because of the letter's better safety profile. It is difficult to imagine there still is an application for MAO inhibitors, except in the rare depression that does not respond to treatment. In the latter cases, my experience is that often medication has not been administered long enough or prescribed in the right dose. Quite frequently there has been no or only inadequate psychotherapy. It is worth remembering that psychotherapy is still and will always be the core treatment for what were a century ago referred to the 'neurotic' conditions, such as reactive depression, anxiety, OCD and the like. The reason is that the symptomatology can be traced to problems in interactions, communication and human relationships. Generally, there is better empirical evidence for the usefulness of antidepressants in the treatment of depression that is chronic (dysthymia) or severe.

In any case, it can take weeks for the full effect of medication to be noticed. A 2008 review of randomized controlled trials concluded that symptomatic improvement with SSRIs was greatest by the end of the first week of use, but that some improvement continued for at least 6 weeks.

Major depressive disorder

The UK National Institute for Health and Care Excellence (NICE) 2009 guidelines indicate that antidepressants should not be routinely used for the initial treatment of mild depression, because the risk-benefit ratio is poor. The guidelines recommend that antidepressant treatment should be considered for:

- People with a history of moderate or severe depression,
- Those with mild depression that has been present for a long period,
- As a second-line treatment for mild depression that persists after other interventions,

- As a first-line treatment for moderate or severe depression.

The guidelines further note that antidepressant treatment should be used in combination with psychosocial interventions in most cases, should be continued for at least 6 months to reduce the risk of relapse, and that SSRIs are typically better tolerated than other antidepressants.

Non-Responders

Between 30% and 50% of individuals treated with a given antidepressant do not show a response. In clinical studies, approximately one-third of patients achieve a full remission, one-third experience a response and one-third are non-responders. Partial remission is characterized by the presence of poorly defined residual symptoms. These symptoms typically include depressed mood, psychic anxiety, sleep disturbance, fatigue and diminished interest or pleasure. It is currently unclear which factors predict partial remission. However, residual symptoms are powerful predictors of relapse, with relapse rates 3–6 times higher in patients with residual symptoms than in those who experience full remission.

"Trial and error" switching

The American Psychiatric Association 2000 Practice Guideline advises that where no response is achieved following six to eight weeks of treatment with an antidepressant, to switch to an antidepressant in the same class, then to a different class of antidepressant. A 2006 meta-analysis review found wide variation in the findings of prior studies; for patients who had failed to respond to an SSRI antidepressant, between 12% and 86% showed a response to a new drug. However, the more antidepressants an individual had already tried, the less likely they were to benefit from a new antidepressant trial. A later meta-analysis found no difference between switching to a new drug and staying on the old medication; although 34% of treatment resistant patients responded when switched to the new drug, 40% responded without being switched.

Combination

A combination strategy involves adding another antidepressant, usually from a different class of antidepressants to have effect on other mechanisms. Although this may be used in clinical practice, there is little evidence for the relative efficacy or adverse effects of this strategy.

Augmentation

For a partial response, the American Psychiatric Association guidelines suggest augmentation, or adding a drug from an altogether different class of substances. These include lithium and thyroid augmentation, dopamine agonists, sex steroids, NRIs, glucocorticoid-specific agents, or the newer anticonvulsants.

An Overview of Psychiatric Medication

Which medication to use?

The medication used needs to be tailored specifically to the individual and the set of effects that are desired and those which need to be voided. However, there seem to be clear favorites overall, which the following list of antidepressant prescriptions in the US in 2010 shows.

Drug Name	Drug Class	Total Prescriptions	Formulations
Sertraline	SSRI	33,409,838	
Citalopram	SSRI	27,993,635	
Fluoxetine	SSRI	24,473,994	
Escitalopram	SSRI	23,000,456	
Trazodone	SARI	18,786,495	
Venlafaxine	SNRI	16,110,606	all formulations
Bupropion	NDRI	15,792,653	al formulations
Duloxetine	SNRI	14,591,949	
Paroxetine	SSRI	12,979,366	
Amitriptyline	TCA	12,611,254	
Venlafaxine XR	SNRI	7,603,949	
Bupropion XL	NDRI	7,317,814	
Mirtazapine	NaSSA / TeCA	6,308,288	
Venlafaxine ER	SNRI	5,526,132	
Bupropion SR	NDRI	4,588,996	
Desvenlafaxine	SNRI	3,412,354	
Nortriptyline	TCA	3,210,476	
Bupropion ER	NDRI	3,132,327	
Venlafaxine	SNRI	2,980,525	
Bupropion	NDRI	753,516	

Psychotherapy

In any case, medication should always be combined with psychotherapy. In the less severe forms of depression and those that seem to have an explanation and are "reactive", medication often shows to be less effective and psychotherapy eventually leads in many cases to a full remission of the symptoms.

Anxiety, Panic Attacks

Introduction

Anxiety is an emotion characterized by an unpleasant state of inner turmoil, often accompanied by nervous behavior, such as pacing back and forth, somatic complaints, and rumination. [1] It is the subjectively unpleasant feelings of dread over anticipated events, such as the feeling of imminent death. [2]

Anxiety vs Fear

Anxiety is not the same as fear, which is a response to a real or perceived immediate threat, [3] whereas anxiety is the expectation of future threat. [3] Anxiety is a feeling of uneasiness and worry, usually generalized and unfocused as an overreaction to a situation that is only subjectively seen as menacing. [4] It is often accompanied by muscular tension, [3] restlessness, fatigue and problems in concentration. Anxiety can be appropriate, but when experienced regularly the individual may suffer from an anxiety disorder. [3]

Diversity of Anxiety

People facing anxiety may withdraw from situations which have provoked anxiety in the past. [5] There are various types of anxiety. Existential anxiety can occur when a person faces angst, an existential crisis, or nihilistic feelings. People can also face mathematical anxiety, somatic anxiety, stage fright, or test anxiety. Social anxiety and stranger anxiety are caused when people are apprehensive around strangers or other people in general. Furthermore, anxiety has been linked with physical symptoms such as IBS and can heighten other mental health illnesses such as OCD and panic disorder. The first step in the management of a person with anxiety symptoms is to evaluate the possible presence of an underlying medical cause, whose recognition is essential in order to decide its correct treatment. [6][7] Anxiety symptoms may be masking an organic disease or appear associated or as a result of a medical disorder. [6][7][8][9]

Duration

Anxiety can be either a short term "state" or a long term "trait". Whereas trait anxiety represents worrying about future events, anxiety disorders are a group of mental disorders characterized by feelings of anxiety and fear. [10] Anxiety disorders are partly genetic but may also be due to drug use, including alcohol, caffeine, and benzodiazepines (which are often prescribed to treat anxiety), as well as withdrawal from drugs of abuse. They often occur with other mental disorders, particularly bipolar disorder, eating disorders, major depressive disorder, or certain personality disorders. Common treatment options include lifestyle changes, medication, and therapy.

Treatment: Psychotherapy and long-term medication

In general medicine, there is still a reflex to prescribe only short-term medication for symptoms of anxiety and panic attacks. While anxiolytics have their place in the treatment of anxiety and panic attacks, especially in reducing the patient's anxiety about having anxiety of panic attacks in the future, they should be an add-on to a combination of psychotherapy and long-term medication, such as an antidepressant from the group of selective serotonin reuptake inhibitors (SSRIs).

Risk Factors for Anxiety

Neuroanatomy

Highly relevant for anxiety is probably the neural circuitry involving the amygdala, which regulates emotions like anxiety and fear and stimulates the hypothalamic-pituitary-adrenal (HPA) Axis and the sympathetic nervous system, and the hippocampus, which is implicated in emotional memory along with the amygdala. People who have anxiety tend to show high activity in response to emotional stimuli in the amygdala. Some writers believe that excessive anxiety can lead to an overpotentiation of the limbic system (which includes the amygdala and nucleus accumbens), giving increased future anxiety, but this does not appear to have been proven.

Research upon adolescents who as infants had been highly apprehensive, vigilant, and fearful finds that their nucleus accumbens is more sensitive than that in other people when deciding to make an action that determined whether they received a reward. This suggests a link between circuits responsible for fear and also reward in anxious people. As researchers note, "a sense of 'responsibility', or self-agency, in a context of uncertainty (probabilistic outcomes) drives the neural system underlying appetitive motivation (i.e., nucleus accumbens) more strongly in temperamentally inhibited than noninhibited adolescents".

Genetic

Genetics and family history (e.g., parental anxiety) may predispose an individual for an increased risk of an anxiety disorder, but generally external stimuli will trigger its onset or exacerbation. Genetic differences account for about 43% of variance in panic disorder and 28% in generalized anxiety disorder. Although single genes are neither necessary nor sufficient for anxiety by themselves, several gene polymorphisms have been found to correlate with anxiety: PLXNA2, SERT, CRH, COMT and BDNF. Several of these genes influence neurotransmitters (such as serotonin and norepinephrine) and hormones (such as cortisol) which are implicated in anxiety. The epigenetic signature of at least one of these genes BDNF has also been associated with anxiety and specific patterns of neural activity.

Medical conditions

Many medical conditions can cause anxiety. This includes conditions that affect the ability to breathe, like COPD and asthma, and the difficulty in breathing that often occurs near death. Conditions that cause abdominal pain or chest pain can cause anxiety and may in some cases be a somatization of anxiety; the same is true for some sexual dysfunctions. Conditions that affect the face or the skin can cause social anxiety especially among adolescents, and developmental disabilities often lead to social anxiety for children as well. Life-threatening conditions like cancer also cause anxiety.

Furthermore, certain organic diseases may present with anxiety or symptoms that mimic anxiety. These disorders include certain endocrine diseases (hypo- and hyperthyroidism, hyperprolactinemia), metabolic disorders (diabetes), deficiency states (low levels of vitamin D, B2, B12, folic acid), gastrointestinal diseases (celiac disease, non-celiac gluten sensitivity, inflammatory bowel disease), heart diseases, blood diseases (anemia), cerebral vascular accidents (transient ischemic attack, stroke), and brain degenerative diseases (Parkinson's disease, dementia, multiple sclerosis, Huntington's disease), among others.

Substance-induced

Several drugs can cause or worsen anxiety, whether in intoxication, withdrawal, or from chronic use. These include alcohol, tobacco, cannabis, sedatives (including prescription benzodiazepines), opioids (including prescription pain killers and illicit drugs like heroin), stimulants (such as caffeine, cocaine and amphetamines), hallucinogens, and inhalants. While many often report self-medicating anxiety with these substances, improvements in anxiety from drugs are usually short-lived (with worsening of anxiety in the long-term, sometimes with acute anxiety as soon as the drug effects wear off) and tend to be exaggerated. Acute exposure to toxic levels of benzene may cause euphoria, anxiety, and irritability lasting up to 2 weeks after the exposure.

Psychological

Poor coping skills (e.g., rigidity/inflexible problem solving, denial, avoidance, impulsivity, extreme self-expectation, affective instability, and inability to focus on problems) are associated with anxiety. Anxiety is also linked and perpetuated by the person's own pessimistic outcome expectancy and how they cope with feedback negativity. Temperament (e.g., neuroticism) and attitudes (e.g. pessimism) have been found to be risk factors for anxiety.

Cognitive distortions such as overgeneralizing, catastrophizing, mind reading, emotional reasoning, binocular trick, and mental filter can result in anxiety. For example, an overgeneralized belief that something bad "always" happens may lead someone to have excessive fears of even minimally risky situations and to avoid benign social situations due to anticipatory anxiety of embarrassment. Such unhealthy thoughts can be targets for successful treatment with cognitive therapy.

Psychodynamic theory posits that anxiety is often the result of opposing unconscious wishes or fears that manifest via maladaptive defense mechanisms (such as suppression, repression, anticipation, regression, somatization, passive aggression, dissociation) that develop to adapt to problems with early objects (e.g., caregivers) and empathic failures in childhood. For example, persistent parental discouragement of anger may result in repression/suppression of angry feelings which manifests as gastrointestinal distress (somatization) when provoked by another while the anger remains unconscious and outside the individual's awareness. Such conflicts can be targets for successful treatment with psychodynamic therapy.

Evolutionary psychology

An evolutionary psychology explanation is that increased anxiety serves the purpose of increased vigilance regarding potential threats in the environment as well as increased tendency to take proactive actions regarding such possible threats. This may cause false positive reactions but an individual suffering from anxiety may also avoid real threats. This may explain why anxious people are less likely to die due to accidents.

When people are confronted with unpleasant and potentially harmful stimuli such as foul odors or tastes, PET-scans show increased blood flow in the amygdala. In these studies, the participants also reported moderate anxiety. This might indicate that anxiety is a protective mechanism designed to prevent the organism from engaging in potentially harmful behaviors.

Social

Social risk factors for anxiety include a history of trauma (e.g., physical, sexual or emotional abuse or assault), early life experiences and parenting factors (e.g., rejection, lack of warmth, high hostility, harsh discipline, high maternal negative affect, anxious childrearing, modelling of dysfunctional and drug-abusing behavior, discouragement of emotions, poor socialization, poor attachment, and child abuse and neglect), cultural factors (e.g., stoic families/cultures, persecuted minorities including the disabled), and socioeconomics (e.g., uneducated, unemployed, impoverished (although developed countries have higher rates of anxiety disorders than developing countries)).One problem with benzodiazepines is that they can be addictive and lead to withdrawal symptoms, although there is some discussion whether they are addictive in their own right or only in association with some other predisposing factors or negative behaviors. This is the reason why they are often only recommended for short term use. However, often an anxious patient can be helped by just carrying the tablet in his/her pocket. And benzodiazepines still play an important role in the treatment of anxieties and panic attacks. They are also used if first-line sleep medication, such as a sleep-inducing antidepressant or a z-drug in the short run, is not effective enough.

Medication

Benzodiazepines

Most anxiolytics belong to the group of benzodiazepines, and although they can be very effective in reducing anxiety for up to a couple of hours, they have three main disadvantages.

The first disadvantage is that they are potentially addictive if taken regularly, the second that they do not work instantaneously, and their effect only lasts for a short time, and the third that they can lead to drowsiness and a lowered reaction time, which means that a patient on this medication should not be driving a car or operating heavy machinery while taking them. If someone suffers from sudden anxiety bouts of anxiety or even panic attacks, it can be over by the time the medication starts working. However, many patients are helped quite effectively by merely having an anxiolytic in their pocket. This works because often the anxiety about feeling anxious and having all the physical symptoms associated with it is the main factor in maintaining the anxiety.

Some common benzodiazepines include:

> Alprazolam (Xanax®), anxiolytic
> Chlordiazepoxide (Librium®), anxiolytic
> Clonazepam (Klonopin®), anxiolytic
> Diazepam (Valium®), anxiolytic
> Lorazepam (Ativan®), anxiolytic
> Nitrazepam (Mogadon®), hypnotic
> Temazepam (Restoril®), hypnotic

Non-benzodiazepine anxiolytics

There are alternatives to the benzodiazepines. However, drugs like buspiron (Buspar®), can take weeks to unfold their anxiolytic effect and many patients do not find them as effective as the benzodiazepines. Often a better option is to start with a benzodiazepine and an SSRI and to wait until the benzodiazepine is no longer needed. For most SSRIs, this interval is in the region of two to three weeks. However, it can be much faster or in some cases even take months.

Selective Serotonin Reuptake Inhibitors (SSRIs)

The long-term solution should be a combination of psychotherapy/counselling and, if indicated, an antidepressant from the group of serotonin reuptake inhibitors (SSRIs). Neurobiologically, all SSRIs can be effective in reducing anxiety and allowing even house bound patients to partake in daily life again, but a few of them are usually prescribed in practice. While they can take up to three weeks, and sometimes even more, to show their full effect, they are generally described as non-addictive and especially in the case of the newer ones, such as escitalopram, patients report few, and in many cases no side-effects. If there are mild side-effects, they often tend to go away after a couple of days. In the case of anxiety, starting with a very low dose (a quarter tablet) for two days and then increasing the dose slowly mostly eliminates subjective side-effects. In practice, if there are side effects in the beginning in the form of tension and an increase in anxiety, this often actually means that they will work. The side effects probably come from the increased serotonin levels at the synapses meeting a hypersensitivity to serotonin. A reconfiguration in the receptor density takes time but will lead to a fading away of the symptoms and the heightened anxiety levels.

The mainstream opinion is that they can be taken over many years and are quite safe. One should pick the SSRI with the best side effect profile for the specific patients. Escitalopram, for example, is linked less with weight gain and nervousness. Sertraline can be more activating, citalopram and paroxetine more sedating. Paroxetine can be increased in dose to 60mg if OCD is also an issue. Higher doses of fluoxetine and sertraline can also be helpful if an eating disorder is a comorbid problem. However, at least in theory, in different doses all the SSRIs can have similar effects.

SSRIs can be combined with a variety of other drugs. However, they should not be combined with MAO inhibitors (antidepressants), certain neuroleptics and other medication, which can increase the serotonin level and in combination lead to the rare but potentially life-threatening serotonin syndrome. They can increase the effect of alcohol, so additional care should be taken in this regard.

Being for at least six months to a year on SSRIs often seems to have the effect, that once the medication is discontinued anxieties are less likely to return for some time. The reason does not seem to be entirely biological but also an effect of learning. As the memory of feeling anxious becomes a distant memory, one is less likely to feel anxious.

Before an SSRI is given certain conditions should be excluded in a conversation with the patient. Among them are a certain type of heart arrhythmia (abnormalities in the QT interval). If the patient is treated for a medical condition, it helps contacting the GP or specialist and asking if there are any indications the patient might suffer from a condition that may be a reason for caution.

But overall, the SSRIs, with escitalopram as a personal favorite, have shown to be an enormous help in treating anxiety and allowing patients to lead normal lives. In combination with psychotherapy / counselling the long-term prognosis for anxiety disorders in most cases has become very good.

References

1. Seligman, M.E.P.; Walker, E.F.; Rosenhan, D.L. Abnormal psychology (4th ed.). New York: W.W. Norton & Company.

2. Davison, Gerald C. (2008). Abnormal Psychology. Toronto: Veronica Visentin. p. 154. ISBN 978-0-470-84072-6.

3. American Psychiatric Association (2013). Diagnostic and Statistical Manual of Mental Disorders (Fifth ed.). Arlington, VA: American Psychiatric Publishing. p. 189. ISBN 978-0-89042-555-8.

4. Bouras, N.; Holt, G. (2007). Psychiatric and Behavioral Disorders in Intellectual and Developmental Disabilities (2nd ed.). Cambridge University Press.

5. Barker, P. (2003). Psychiatric and Mental Health Nursing: The Craft of Caring. London: Edward Arnold. ISBN 978-0-340-81026-2.

6. World Health Organization (2009). Pharmacological Treatment of Mental Disorders in Primary Health Care (PDF). Geneva. ISBN 978-92-4-154769-7.

7. Testa A, Giannuzzi R, Daini S, Bernardini L, Petrongolo L, Gentiloni Silveri N (2013). "Psychiatric emergencies (part III): psychiatric symptoms resulting from organic diseases" (PDF). Eur Rev Med Pharmacol Sci (Review). 17 Suppl 1: 86–99.

8. Testa A, Giannuzzi R, Sollazzo F, Petrongolo L, Bernardini L, Daini S (2013). "Psychiatric emergencies (part II): psychiatric disorders coexisting with organic diseases." (PDF). Eur Rev Med Pharmacol Sci. 17 (Suppl 1): 65–85. PMID 23436668.

9. Testa A, Giannuzzi R, Sollazzo F, Petrongolo L, Bernardini L, Daini S (2013). "Psychiatric emergencies (part I): psychiatric disorders

causing organic symptoms."(PDF). Eur Rev Med Pharmacol Sci. 17 (Suppl 1): 55–64. PMID 23436668.

10. Diagnostic and Statistical Manual of Mental DisordersAmerican Psychiatric Associati. (5th ed.). Arlington: American Psychiatric Publishing. 2013. pp. 189–195. ISBN 978-0890425558.

Obsessive Compulsive Disorder (OCD)

Introduction

Psychotherapy is the first line of treatment when it comes to Obsessive Compulsive Disorder (OCD). However, psychotherapy alone is often not enough, especially when a patient is so affected by the condition that leaving the home is no longer possible. Also, medication can be helpful in the beginning of therapy to reduce the level of anxiety and facilitate psychotherapy. It just needs to be pointed out that medication usually takes a significant while to work, frequently months, and in some cases even half a year to a year. One reason is that OCD is to a substantial part learned behavior which requires time to 'unlearn'.

If obsessive thoughts and/or compulsive behaviors interfere with life to an extent that its quality is noticeably reduced, then there is often a strong case for medication. Difficulties in relationships or at the workplace should be a clear signal that the OCD is no longer under control. They can also contribute to the underlying emotional conflicts that maintain the condition, and thus make it worse.

OCD affects people's life severely. It can make it impossible to leave the apartment, work and have a relationship. The patient focuses almost exclusively on thoughts and questions that cannot be resolved or answered. Often the thoughts are about issues that are unclear and uncertain, maybe about distant memories or ruminations or about another person's thoughts. The patient perceives a special relevance in them, which often seems out of proportion to an outside, which in psychotherapy can be addressed quite effectively by shifting the focus to his or her own wants, desire, wishes, aspirations and values. Quite often an emotional conflict between what patients feel they should do and what they want to do maintains the OCD.

There is significant evidence that certain areas in the brain and particular neurotransmitter systems, including serotonin and dopamine, are involved in the maintenance of OCD. Since the brain is a complex networked system where pathways interrelate and affect each other, it is difficult to say which neurotransmitter system and which morphological pathways are more primary in the chain of causation that ultimately leads to OCD. However, given the high plasticity of the nervous system and the enormous volumes of information that reach the brain, are processed by it and sent back out again, small variations in the network and in cellular functioning can lead to significant variations in such higher cognitive functions as recurrent thoughts and thoughts that induce other thoughts, in short, the thought patterns one uses and engages in.

Medication can support the autoregulatory mechanisms of the brain and lead to a reduction in obsessive thoughts and the urge to carry out compulsions, as well lessen the anxiety patients experience when they try to suppress their obsessive thoughts or compulsive behaviors. It is not exactly understood how this works but effects on both, the systems that make some people more predisposed towards OCD like thoughts and behaviors and those that mediate anxiety, seems plausible. In any case, the effects from medication are particularly slow in the case of OCD, often much more so than in the treatment of anxiety and depression, but if patients know this, thy are often more willing to accept the mostly mild and transient side effects that may occur in the first days or weeks.

From Anxiety to OCD

Selective serotonin reuptake inhibitors (SSRIs) seem to work because they reduce the anxiety that maintains the OCD and resurfaces if one tries to suppress intrusive thoughts or compulsive behaviors. SSRIs are usually tried first because they act predominantly on the serotonin system and have relatively safe side-effect profiles, but this does not mean that the effect is not also the result of pathways involving other neurotransmitter systems, as already mentioned.

Reducing anxiety with medication can make it easier for psychotherapeutic approaches, such as CBT or psychodynamic psychotherapy, to help the patient not to engage with the OCD thoughts and not to carry out the compulsive behaviors.

SSRIs as First-Line Treatment

Effective medication is primarily from the class of selective serotonin reuptake inhibitors (SSRIs), which increase the intrasynaptic levels of the neurotransmitter serotonin and thereby change the density of various serotonin receptors in the cell membrane. The latter in conjunction with changes in the physiology and morphology of the neuro itself rather than the mere increase in the neurotransmitter seems responsible for the beneficial effect of this type of medication on depression, anxiety, OCD and other conditions. Most 'serotonergic' antidepressants have shown effectiveness in the treatment of OCD.

Paroxetine and Fluoxetine

Various studies have compared the effectiveness of SSRIs in randomized controlled trials (RCTs), but it seems that all SSRIs have a potential effect on OCD. However, there are some substances that are more likely to be used in daily practice than others. While fluoxetine (Prozac®) is used less often nowadays, mainly because it is more likely to cause feelings of numbness and the sense of being 'wrapped in cotton', and paroxetine (Paxil®) has been a stable and reliable candidate over the years, sertraline, and to some degree escitalopram, seem to be used increasingly. The problem with escitalopram is that it is licensed only in relatively moderate dose, and for OCD often higher doses are required.

The Diversity of SSRIs

Generally, all SSRIs can have an effect of OCD, and it is often a matter of individual experience which one prefers. While at the turn of this century there was a preference for paroxetine, this might now be shifting to escitalopram, which is by many patients reported to be better tolerated, and often sertraline, which can be used at the necessary higher doses that escitalopram is not licensed for. Unfortunately, pharmaceutical companies lose interest to expand the indications of a drug, or its dose range, once the patents expired, as in the case of escitalopram. Clinical experience is crucial in any regard, because there are many different 'flavors' of OCD and co-morbidities which cannot be captured adequately by most studies. A drug which is better in treating anxiety may be better in an individual suffering from both, OCD and anxiety, than one that causes activation and thus potentially more tension and nervousness.

The effect of the medication on the intracellular information transmission is likely responsible for the effect of SSRIs on the mentioned mental health conditions. The uneven distribution of receptor subtype in the brain and a host of other factors make the SSRIs quite specific. An increase in appetite associated with some SSRIs more than with others is likely due to the fact that the center in the brain communicating a hunger signal also uses serotonin as a neurotransmitter. In many patients this is an undesired side effect, while in some this may actually be of therapeutic value. A patient suffering from severe OCD and depression may have lost appetite to an extent that an SSRI which is more likely to increase his or her appetite may be desirable.

SSRIs that have been recommended repeatedly are the following:

>   Citalopram (Cipramil®)
>   Escitalopram (Cipralex®)
>   Fluoxetine (Prozac®)
>   Fluvaxamine (Luvox® and Faverin®)
>   Paroxetine (Paxil® and Seroxat®)
>   Sertraline (Lustral® and Zoloft®)

The NICE guidelines for the treatment of OCD now only recommend two of these medications for use in treating children with OCD. These are Sertraline for children aged 6 years and older and Fluvoxamine for children aged 8 years and older. However, there seems to be no theoretical reasons, why, for example, the newer and usually very well tolerated escitalopram should not also be useful in this regard.

Typically, the process of determining the most suited medication for an individual is achieved on a trial-and-error basis. However, to allow its maximum effects to be adequately observed, each medication should be taken for a specified time, usually for at least 12-16 weeks, before seeking out an alternative.

One should, of course, have an eye on potential side effects and contraindications to the SSRIs, such as a large QT prolongation or side effects from SSRIs in the past that did not fade after a few weeks. Any allergic reactions, such as rashes, on one SSRI occur again on a different SSRI.

Sertraline

Sertraline is effective for the treatment of OCD in adults and children. (1) It was better tolerated and, based on intention to treat analysis, performed better than the gold standard of OCD treatment clomipramine. (2) It is generally accepted that the sertraline dosages necessary for the effective treatment of OCD are higher than the usual dosage for depression. (3) The onset of action is also slower for OCD than for depression. (4)

Cognitive behavioral therapy alone was superior to sertraline in both adults and children; however, the best results were achieved using a combination of these treatments. (5)(6)

High Doses

Relatively high doses of SRIs are needed for effectiveness in the treatment of OCD. (16) Studies have found that high dosages of SSRIs above the normally recommended maximums are significantly more effective in OCD treatment than lower dosages (e.g., 250 to 400 mg/day sertraline versus 200 mg/day sertraline). (11)(16) There is a case report of complete remission from OCD for approximately one month following a massive overdose of fluoxetine, an SSRI with a uniquely long duration of action. (18)

Discontinuing SSRIs

Although SSRIs can be stopped quite easily, it is sensible to reduce them gradually. NICE recommend that if the medication has helped, one should continue taking the medication for at least 12 months to ensure your symptoms continue to improve. This makes it also more likely that there will be an often empirically observed protective after-effect after stopping them.

Non-selective serotonin reuptake inhibitors (NSSRIs)

If these medications fail to work, an NSSRI, mostly a tricyclic antidepressant, may be prescribed. However, because it affects a greater variety of neurotransmitters and receptors in the brain, the breadth of potential side is greater. Therefore, the NSSRIs are not first-choice medication for treating OCD.

Tricyclic Antidepressants

Clomipramine

Clomipramine (Anafranil®) is a tricyclic antidepressant that has been used in the past and may be a secondary choice to the SSRIs. The NICE guidelines state Clomipramine should be considered in the treatment of adults with OCD or BDD after an adequate trial of at least one SSRI has been ineffective or poorly tolerated, or if the patient prefers Clomipramine or has had success in using the medication before.

Clomipramine was the first drug that was investigated for and found to be effective in the treatment of OCD. (7)(17) In addition, it was the first drug to be approved by the FDA in the United States for the treatment of OCD. (8) The effectiveness of clomipramine in the treatment of OCD is far greater than that of other TCAs, which are comparatively weak SRIs; a meta-analysis found pre- versus post-treatment effect sizes of 1.55 for clomipramine relative to a range of 0.67 for imipramine and 0.11 for desipramine. (19) In contrast to other TCAs, studies have found that clomipramine and SSRIs have similar effectiveness in the treatment of OCD. (19) However, multiple meta-analyses have found that clomipramine nonetheless retains a significant effectiveness advantage relative to SSRIs. (13) However, the effectiveness advantage for clomipramine has not been apparent in head-to-head comparisons of clomipramine versus SSRIs for OCD, (13) which may also be a consequence of the different methodologies used.

The combination of clomipramine and SSRIs has also been found to be significantly more effective in alleviating OCD symptoms, and clomipramine is commonly used to augment SSRIs for this reason. (8,16)

In addition to serotonin reuptake inhibition, clomipramine is also a mild but clinically significant antagonist of the dopamine D1, D2, and D3 receptors at high concentrations. (9,13) Addition of antipsychotics, which are potent dopamine receptor antagonists, to SSRIs, has been found to significantly augment their effectiveness in the treatment of OCD. (13,14) As such, besides strong serotonin reuptake inhibition, clomipramine at high doses might also block dopamine receptors to treat OCD symptoms, and this could additionally or alternatively be involved in its possible effectiveness advantage over SSRIs. (12,15)

Although clomipramine is similarly or more effective in the treatment of OCD compared to SSRIs, it is greatly inferior to them in terms of tolerability and safety due to its lack of selectivity for the SERT and promiscuous pharmacological activity. (10,13) In addition, clomipramine has high toxicity in overdose and can potentially result in death, whereas death rarely, if ever, occurs with overdose of SSRIs. (10,13) It is for these reasons that clomipramine, in spite of potentially superior effectiveness to SSRIs, is now rarely used as a first-line agent in the treatment of OCD, with SSRIs being used as first-line therapies instead and clomipramine generally being reserved for more severe cases. (10)

Augmentation with a neuroleptic

In very severe cases with intrusive thoughts one can also add a neuroleptic, whereby possible cross interactions should be kept in mind. Generally, one should avoid combinations that can increase the risk of the otherwise very rare serotonin syndrome, which can be life-threatening and requiring intensive care. Also, one needs to be careful with combinations that prolong the QT time. Olanzapine (Zyprexa®) may be the least problematic on the last point, but it also can prolong the QT time.

Psychotherapy

Medication should not be given alone. It should always be used together with psychotherapy, except in cases where this is not possible.

References

1. Geller DA, Biederman J, Stewart SE, Mullin B, Martin A, Spencer T, Faraone SV (2003). "Which SSRI? A meta-analysis of pharmacotherapy trials in pediatric obsessive-compulsive disorder". The American Journal of Psychiatry. 160 (11): 1919–28.

2. Flament MF, Bisserbe JC (1997). "Pharmacologic treatment of obsessive-compulsive disorder: comparative studies". The Journal of Clinical Psychiatry. 58. Suppl 12: 18–22.

3. Math SB, Janardhan Reddy YC (19 July 2007). "Issues In The Pharmacological Treatment of Obsessive-Compulsive Disorder: First-Line Treatment Options for OCD". medscape.com. Retrieved 01 August 2014

4. Blier P, Habib R, Flament MF (2006). "Pharmacotherapies in the management of obsessive-compulsive disorder" (PDF). Can J Psychiatry. 51 (7): 417–30.

5. Pediatric OCD Treatment Study (POTS) Team (2004). "Cognitive-behavior therapy, sertraline, and their combination for children and adolescents with obsessive-compulsive disorder: the Pediatric OCD Treatment Study (POTS) randomized controlled trial". JAMA. 292 (16): 1969–76.

6. Sousa MB, Isolan LR, Oliveira RR, Manfro GG, Cordioli AV (2006). "A randomized clinical trial of cognitive-behavioral group therapy and sertraline in the treatment of obsessive-compulsive disorder". The Journal of Clinical Psychiatry. 67 (7): 1133–9.

7. Joseph Zohar (31 May 2012). Obsessive Compulsive Disorder: Current Science and Clinical Practice. John Wiley & Sons. pp. 19–30, 32, 50, 59. ISBN 978-1-118-30801-1.

8. Robert Hudak; Darin D. Dougherty (17 February 2011). Clinical Obsessive-Compulsive Disorders in Adults and Children. Cambridge University Press. pp. 31–. ISBN 978-1-139-49626-1.

9. Austin LS, Lydiard RB, Ballenger JC, Cohen BM, Laraia MT, Zealberg JJ, Fossey MD, Ellinwood EH (1991). "Dopamine blocking activity of clomipramine in patients with obsessive-compulsive disorder". Biol. Psychiatry. 30 (3): 225–32.

10. Jonathan S. Abramowitz; Dean McKay; Eric A. Storch (12 June 2017). The Wiley Handbook of Obsessive Compulsive Disorders. Wiley. pp. 1076–. ISBN 978-1-118-89025-7.

11. Byerly MJ, Goodman WK, Christensen R (1996). "High doses of sertraline for treatment-resistant obsessive-compulsive disorder". Am J Psychiatry. 153 (9): 1232–3.

12. Hood, Sean; Alderton, Deirdre; Castle, David (2016). "Obsessive–Compulsive Disorder: Treatment and Treatment Resistance". Australasian Psychiatry. 9 (2): 118–127.

13. Hollander E, Kaplan A, Allen A, Cartwright C (2000). "Pharmacotherapy for obsessive-compulsive disorder". Psychiatr. Clin. North Am. 23 (3): 643–56.

14. Dold M, Aigner M, Lanzenberger R, Kasper S (2013). "Antipsychotic augmentation of serotonin reuptake inhibitors in treatment-resistant obsessive-compulsive disorder: a meta-analysis of double-blind, randomized, placebo-controlled trials". Int. J. Neuropsychopharmacol. 16 (3): 557–74.

15. Fontenelle LF, Nascimento AL, Mendlowicz MV, Shavitt RG, Versiani M (2007). "An update on the pharmacological treatment of obsessive-compulsive disorder". Expert Opin Pharmacother. 8 (5): 563–83.

16. Kellner M (2010). "Drug treatment of obsessive-compulsive disorder". Dialogues Clin Neurosci. 12 (2): 187–97. PMC 3181958 Freely accessible.

17. Jose A. Yaryura-Tobias; Fugen A. Neziroglu (1997). Obsessive-compulsive Disorder Spectrum: Pathogenesis, Diagnosis, and Treatment. American Psychiatric Pub. pp. 36–. ISBN 978-0-88048-707-8.

18. Leonard HL, Topol D, Bukstein O, Hindmarsh D, Allen AJ, Swedo SE (1994). "Clonazepam as an augmenting agent in the treatment of childhood-onset obsessive-compulsive disorder". J Am Acad Child Adolesc Psychiatry. 33 (6): 792–4.

19. Eddy KT, Dutra L, Bradley R, Westen D (2004). "A multidimensional meta-analysis of psychotherapy and pharmacotherapy for obsessive-compulsive disorder". Clin Psychol Rev. 24 (8): 1011–30.

Insomnia

Sleep problems affect many people. Especially in our complex and fast paced world remaining thoughts or emotions from the day can occupy us at night. Dealing with stress effectively, such as prioritizing the activities in one's life in line with one's values and interests, can improve sleep considerably. The mental health diagnostic manual DSM-IV defines insomnia as difficulty initiating sleep or maintaining sleep.

Several mental health conditions can also cause sleeplessness. Major depression, PTSD, trauma, anxiety, bipolar disorders, psychosis and many more can cause insomnia. Many organic diseases can also cause insomnia, as can sleep apnea and chronic pain syndromes. In some cases, where no other reason can be found, an idiopathic insomnia may itself be a mental health problem.

The first step is to identify whether there is a sleep problem that requires treatment. People who sleep seven to eight hours usually do not have a problem with lack of sleep. In the case of paradoxical insomnia, although one believes to have a sleep problem, electrophysiological measurements show no sign of a sleep disturbance.

The second step is to identify if there is inadequate sleep hygiene. If there are behaviors that are not conducive to good sleep, they should be addressed first. Some behaviors increase arousal, such as consuming caffeine or nicotine in the evening or at night. Various drugs, legal and illegal, can affect one's sleep greatly. Intense thoughts or emotions can also disturb one's sleep, as do day-time naps or significant irregularities in the daily sleep-wake schedule.

Treatment of insomnia should also always include psychotherapy. It can help reduce the worries about and consequences of sleeplessness, and thereby break the vicious cycle of insomnia. Feeling less anxious about the ability to get a goodnight's sleep often improves one's sleep. Cognitive therapy, CBT, but also psychodynamic approaches can be helpful.

There are several over-the-counter sleep aids available, often with questionable effectiveness. Nonprescription drugs, such as sedating antihistamines, protein precursors, and a host of other substances can work in individual cases, but they are often not strong enough even in cases of moderate insomnia. L-Tryptophan has been withdrawn from the market after it was linked to outbreaks of eosinophilia. Melatonin may help some individuals, although the placebo should not be underestimated.

Most hypnotics are approved by the U.S. Food and Drug Administration (FDA) only for short-term use. The z-drugs zolpidem (Stilnoct®, Ambien®, Ambien CR®, Intermezzo®, Stilnox® and eszopiclone (Lunesta®), as well as the melatonin-receptor agonist ramelteon (Rozerem®) are exceptions. The z-drugs are by their function related to the benzodiazepines and are also considered potentially addictive if taken regularly. This means that if they are stopped one's sleep might be worse for a while. There could also be an additional increase in anxiety and, at least theoretically, panic attacks. Benzodiazepines and z-drugs should not be used while driving a car or operating heavy machinery, and the longer lasting ones can lead to a hangover in the morning and drowsiness during the day.

If the insomnia has lasted for a while and is expected to reoccur for at least a couple of weeks, sleep inducing antidepressants should be considered first choice. Mirtazapine (Remeron®) is often a good option, which in clinical experience is more sleep inducing at lower doses (15mg) than at higher doses (45mg). Second-generation antipsychotics, such as Olanzapine (Zyprexa®) are also used, but it seems there should be some other symptom or reason that justifies their use because of the potentially more serious die-effects. If the insomnia is combined with some types of obsessive thoughts or even Tourette's syndrome, for example, sleep inducing second-generation antipsychotics may be a logical choice.

Psychotherapeutic treatment of insomnia is discussed in my other articles, but medication as a supportive measure seems warranted in some cases, especially if a modern antidepressant can help the patient maintain a job or a relationship, while using therapy to explore the reasons of the sleep disturbance.

Listed below are some substances that are used to treat insomnia.

We will start with the group of benzodiazepines and then move on to the pharmacologically closely related z-drugs, which should usually be preferred to the former, if they are used at all.

Benzodiazepines

The most commonly used class of hypnotics for insomnia are the benzodiazepines. Benzodiazepines are not significantly better for insomnia than antidepressants. [1] While they have an important role in anxiety and panic attacks, especially in the time interval until an antidepressant works, their role in the treatment of insomnia should only occur in niche cases, and only over a short internal. The z-drugs, which also work on the benzodiazepine receptor should be preferred, if at all necessary. In clinical practice, the risk for dependency seems higher if the benzodiazepines are used as sleeping pills than if they are used in acute anxiety attacks.

Benzodiazepines all bind unselectively to the GABA-A receptor. There is some indication that certain benzodiazepines (hypnotic benzodiazepines) have significantly higher activity at the α1 subunit of the GABA-A receptor compared to other benzodiazepines (for example, triazolam and temazepam have significantly higher activity at the α1 subunit compared to alprazolam and diazepam, making them superior sedative-hypnotics – alprazolam and diazepam, in turn, have higher activity at the α2 subunit compared to triazolam and temazepam, making them superior anxiolytic agents). Modulation of the α1 subunit is associated with sedation, motor impairment, respiratory depression, amnesia, ataxia, and reinforcing behavior (drug-seeking behavior). Modulation of the α2 subunit is associated with anxiolytic activity and disinhibition. For this reason, certain benzodiazepines may be better suited to treat insomnia than others.

>Triazolam (Halcion®)
>Temazepam (Restoril®)
>[Alprazolam (Xanax®)]

and others may be useful as an insomnia medication that stays in the system longer. For instance, they have been effectively used to treat sleep problems such as sleepwalking and night terrors. However, these drugs may cause sleepiness during the day and can also cause tolerance.

Chronic use

With chronic use, the sleep-inducing effect of the benzodiazepines often goes away, while the risk of tolerance increases quite quickly if they are used as hypnotics. Chronic users of hypnotic medications have more regular nighttime awakenings than patients suffering from insomnia who are not taking hypnotic medications. (2) Hypnotics should be prescribed for only a few days at the lowest effective dose and avoided altogether wherever possible, especially in the elderly. (3) Between 1993 and 2010, the prescribing of benzodiazepines to individuals with sleep disorders has decreased from 24% to 11% in the US, coinciding with the first release of nonbenzodiazepines. (4)

Common Side Effects

The benzodiazepine and nonbenzodiazepine hypnotic medications have a number of side-effects such as day time fatigue, changes in reaction time potentially leading to motor vehicle crashes and other accidents, cognitive impairments and falls and fractures. Elderly people are more sensitive to these side-effects. (5)

Some benzodiazepines have demonstrated effectiveness in sleep maintenance in the short term but in the longer-term benzodiazepines can lead to tolerance, physical dependence, benzodiazepine withdrawal syndrome upon discontinuation, and long-term worsening of sleep, especially after consistent usage over long periods of time. Benzodiazepines, while inducing unconsciousness, actually worsen sleep as—like alcohol—they promote light sleep while decreasing time spent in deep sleep. (6) A further problem is, with regular use of short-acting sleep aids for insomnia, daytime rebound anxiety can emerge. (7)

Although there is little evidence for benefit of benzodiazepines in insomnia compared to other treatments and evidence of major harm, prescriptions have continued to increase. (8) This is likely due to their addictive nature, both due to misuse and because—through their rapid action, tolerance and withdrawal—they can "trick" insomniacs into thinking they are helping with sleep. There is a general awareness that long-term use of benzodiazepines for insomnia in most people is inappropriate and that a gradual withdrawal is usually beneficial due to the adverse effects associated with the long-term use of benzodiazepines and is recommended whenever possible. (9)

Z-Drugs

Zolpidem (Ambien®, Intermezzo®)

They often work quite well, but some patients wake up in the middle of the night. Zolpidem is now available in an extended release version, Ambien CR®. This helps prolong the effect of the medication. The FDA has approved a prescription oral spray called Zolpimist®, which contains zolpidem, for the short-term treatment of insomnia brought on by difficulty falling asleep.

Eszopiclone (Lunesta®)

Studies show people sleep an average of seven to eight hours. Because of the risk of impairment, the next day, the FDA recommends the starting dose of Lunesta® be no more than 1 mg.

Zaleplon (Sonata®)

Zaleplon stays active in the body for the shortest amount of time. That means patients can try to fall asleep on their own. Then, if they are still not asleep at 2 a.m., they can take it without feeling drowsy in the morning. However, if one tends to wake during the night, this might not be the best choice.

Melatonin-receptor agonist

Ramelteon (Rozerem®)

This is a sleep medication that works differently than the others. It works by targeting the sleep-wake cycle, not by depressing the central nervous system. It is prescribed for people who have difficulty falling asleep. Rozerem® can be prescribed for long-term use, and the drug has so far shown no evidence of abuse or dependence.

Antidepressants

Mirtazapine (Remeron®)

Lower doses (15 mg) are often effective in inducing sleep, while higher doses (30-45 mg) have a greater antidepressant effectiveness, though may be less beneficial for sleep. Unfortunately, an increase in appetite and weight gain frequently requires a switch to a different antidepressant, such as trazodone, which seems less associated with this side effect.

Doxepine (Silenor®)

This tricyclic antidepressant is approved for use in people who have trouble staying asleep. Silenor® may help with sleep maintenance by blocking histamine receptors. Dosage is based on health, age, and response to therapy. Caution is required with all the tricyclic antidepressants as they can prolong the QT interval and have a number of other potentially severe side-effects.

Trazodone (Desyrel®)

Trazodone is an antidepressant, which is less effective as an antidepressant, but often helpful in inducing sleep.

Antipsychotics

Certain antipsychotic drugs like Olanzapin (Zyprexa®) also have a sedative effect and they are sometimes used in slow doses as sleep medication. However, because of the rare but potentially severe side-effects of neuroleptics, even in the second generation, they should not be used as sleep medication without any other rational for using them.

Over-the-Counter Sleep Aids

Most of these sleeping pills are antihistamines. They generally work well but can cause some drowsiness the next day. They are generally considered safe enough to be sold without a prescription. However, if combined with other drugs that also contain antihistamines, like cold or allergy medications, one could inadvertently take too much.

Sleep medication can have a number of side-effects. In 2007, the FDA issued warnings for prescription sleep drugs, alerting patients that they can cause rare allergic reactions and complex sleep-related behaviors, including "sleep driving." Medication should in the case of a sleeping disorder always be the last option. Better sleep hygiene and psychotherapy/counselling should come long before it and be the first choice. No sleeping pill can take away worries about the job or one's relationship or correct for drinking coffee in the evening or sleeping next to one's laptop.

References

1. Buscemi, N.; Vandermeer, B.; Friesen, C.; Bialy, L.; Tubman, M.; Ospina, M.; Klassen, T. P.; Witmans, M. (2007). "The Efficacy and Safety of Drug Treatments for Chronic Insomnia in Adults: A Meta-analysis of RCTs". Journal of General Internal Medicine. 22 (9): 1335–1350. doi:10.1007/s11606-007-0251-z. PMID 17619935.

2. Ohayon, M. M.; Caulet, M. (1995). "Insomnia and psychotropic drug consumption". Progress in neuro-psychopharmacology & biological psychiatry. 19 (3): 421–431. doi:10.1016/0278-5846(94)00023-B. PMID 7624493.

3. "What's wrong with prescribing hypnotics?". Drug and therapeutics bulletin. 42 (12): 89–93. 2004. doi:10.1136/dtb.2004.421289. PMID 15587763.

4. Kaufmann, Christopher N.; Spira, Adam P.; Alexander, G. Caleb; Rutkow, Lainie; Mojtabai, Ramin (2015). "Trends in prescribing of sedative-hypnotic medications in the USA: 1993–2010". Pharmacoepidemiology and Drug Safety. 25: 637–45. doi:10.1002/pds.3951. ISSN 1099-1557. PMID 26711081.

5. Glass, J.; Lanctôt, K. L.; Herrmann, N.; Sproule, B. A.; Busto, U. E. (2005). "Sedative hypnotics in older people with insomnia: Meta-analysis of risks and benefits". BMJ. 331 (7526): 1169. doi:10.1136/bmj.38623.768588.47. PMID 16284208.

6. Tsoi, W. F. (1991). "Insomnia: Drug treatment". Annals of the Academy of Medicine, Singapore. 20 (2): 269–272. PMID 1679317.

7. Montplaisir, J. (2000). "Treatment of primary insomnia". Canadian Medical Association Journal. 163 (4): 389–391. PMC 80369Freely accessible. PMID 10976252.

8. Carlstedt, Roland A. (13 December 2009). Handbook of Integrative Clinical Psychology, Psychiatry, and Behavioral Medicine: Perspectives, Practices, and Research. Springer. pp. 128–130. ISBN 0-8261-1094-0.

9. Authier, N.; Boucher, A.; Lamaison, D.; Llorca, P. M.; Descotes, J.; Eschalier, A. (2009). "Second Meeting of the French CEIP (Centres d'Évaluation et d'Information sur la Pharmacodépendance). Part II: Benzodiazepine Withdrawal". Thérapie. 64 (6): 365–370.

Bipolar Disorder

Basic Treatments

Bipolar disorder is a condition that can be treated with a combination of medication and psychotherapy/counselling. Especially the less severe forms often remain untreated, leading to unnecessary suffering, also in terms of failed relationships and absences at the workplace, and even suicide. Treatment should always include psychotherapy. Research shows that people who take medication for bipolar disorder tend to recover much faster and control their moods better if they also get therapy.

Medication with mood stabilizers can bring mania and depression under control and prevent relapses once the mood has stabilized. Medication should be regarded as long-term treatment. In many cases, medication is not used long enough, leading to a relapse that interferes significantly with the quality of life or even suicidal thoughts. Sometimes, stopping the medication may be necessary due to side effects or other reasons, Lamotrigine (e.g. Lamictal®), for example, quite frequently causes skin rashes, which, though they do so rarely, can lead into the potentially fatal Stevens-Johnson syndrome, a condition with necrotic skin lesions. However, in the clear majority of cases, mood stabilizers are tolerated well and can help the patient to lead a normal private and professional life.

Psychotherapy as a complement helps individuals with bipolar disorder to get a better sense of themselves, their needs, wants and values, to acquire strategies to reduce stress and anxiety, and to increase their influence over the depths and heights of the mood swings. Since mood depends on thoughts, activities and situations as well as sleep hygiene and caring for one's physical health, there is a lot that can be done besides medication, which nevertheless remains the most important piece of treatment for bipolar disorder.

Making healthy choices in one's life can affect mental-wellbeing. Alcohol is a depressant and makes recovery even more difficult. It can also interfere with the way medication works.

Long-Term Medication

Medication should be continued over a while, even if the bipolar symptoms disappear, because of the high rate of relapse after discontinuing medication. Therapy probably can reduce the risk to a degree, but it is important not to discontinue the medication too early. Most mood stabilizers can take a long time to bring about a notable difference in the patient. Antipsychotics can work faster, while lithium can take months or even half a year to show a satisfactory effect. The effect from ending medication may also not be felt for a while, especially in cases where the mood swings were triggered by certain events or stressors, which would need to reoccur to be able to judge if the bipolar condition went into remission and there is no longer a need for mood stabilizing medication.

Individualized Medication

It can take a while to find the right bipolar medication and dose. Everyone responds to medication differently, so it may be necessary to try some before settling on one that has the best trade-off between high effectiveness and low side-effects.

Patients with bipolar disorder should be seen more often when medication with bipolar drugs is begun. There should be room for support and therapy to help with anxieties, doubts, social, work-related and partnership problems and questions in general. During acute mania or depression, most patients talk with their healthcare professional at least once a week, or even every day, to monitor symptoms, medication doses, and side effects. Once the symptoms have subsided, medical monitoring can gradually be done less frequently, although it is still good practice to see patients once per quarter as a minimum. They should also be told to make contact quickly if they have suicidal or violent feelings, changes in mood, sleep, or energy or changes in medication side effects.

Comprehensive Consultation

Since medication used to treat bipolar disorder can have interactions with other drugs, whether over-the-counter or prescribed, this should be discussed. Possible interactions with other medication, side-effects that can affect one's ability to drive or operate machinery and the risks for pregnancy should be discussed. Using a daily reminder/medication saver system can be helpful. Also, it is important to inform patients about the monitoring that may have to be done, such as the need for frequent blood works in the case of lithium, especially early in treatment, after changing the dose or if there are circumstances that effect how the medication works and/or its metabolism

Diagnosis

An accurate diagnosis is important, especially in distinguishing between monopolar depression and bipolar disorders. Antidepressants can trigger manic episodes especially if there already is an underlying bipolar disorder. If they are needed to treat the depressive episodes in a bipolar disorder, they should only be used in combination with a mood stabilizer to prevent the exacerbation of a manic episode.

Mood Stabilizers

In the following, some important mood stabilizers used in the treatment of bipolar disorders are discussed. Mood stabilizers are medications that help control the highs and lows of bipolar disorder. They are the cornerstone of treatment, both for mania and depression. Chemically and functionally the family of antidepressants is very diverse. Unlike the serotonin hypothesis in depression, there have never been widely accepted general theories for the pathogenesis of bipolar disorder.

- Lithium
- Anticonvulsants
- Antipsychotics

Benzodiazepines
Calcium channel blockers
Thyroid hormone

Lithium

Lithium was the first mood stabilizer for bipolar disorder Lithium is the oldest and most well-known mood stabilizer. It is highly effective for treating mania but can also help in the treatment of bipolar depression. It is not as effective for mixed episodes or rapid cycling forms of bipolar disorder. Often patients notice greater stability in their mood swings early on, full effectiveness, however, can take up to a couple of months.

The following side effects are common on lithium. Some may go away as the body adapts to the medication.

- Weight gain
- Drowsiness
- Tremor
- Weakness or fatigue
- Excessive thirst; increased urination
- Stomach pain
- Thyroid problems
- Memory and concentration problems
- Nausea, vertigo
- Diarrhea

Regular blood tests are necessary to make sure the blood levels are within a narrow therapeutic window. A dose that is too high can be toxic, one that is too low ineffective. Ranges for blood levels can vary from lab to lab, hospital to hospital and country to country. The lowest seems to be 0.4 mmol/L and the upper limit 1.2 mmol/L. However, it is always important to remember that ultimately the patient's symptoms are treated and not the blood lithium level. I have seen 0.5 a perfectly sufficient dose in some cases, while in others 1.1 was needed. The famous lithium tremor may be one of the earliest signs when one reaches toxic levels, but there is no guarantee it always will be. I would start out with weekly lithium blood levels, and after reaching a stable dose to biweekly tests. After about six weeks one can move to monthly tests. In most cases, if one stays within a therapeutic range with 1.2 mmol/L as the upper limit and conducts regular blood tests, lithium is relatively safe and effective.

After the first couple of months and if the medication works well and side-effects are either tolerable or absent, the frequency of blood tests may be reduced to every two to three months. But it should not be discontinued completely because various changes in eating habits, athletic activities and other medication can affect the lithium blood levels.

Other factors that can influence the lithium levels are:

> Weight loss or gain
> The amount of sodium in the diet
> Seasonal changes (lithium levels may be higher in the summer)
> Many prescription and over-the-counter drugs (e.g. ibuprofen, diuretics, and heart and blood pressure medication)
> Caffeine, tea, and coffee
> Dehydration

Hormonal fluctuations during the menstrual cycle and pregnancy

Changes in health (for example, heart disease and kidney disease increase the risk of lithium toxicity)

The amount of salt in the diet should not suddenly be changed; it is especially important not to suddenly reduce your salt intake. Patients should make sure that they drink enough fluids, especially if one exercises heavily or in hot weather when one will sweat more. Alcoholic drinks can lead to an overall water loss, which can become a problem especially in hot weather of when one tries to still one's thirst by drinking alcoholic beverages.

Anticonvulsants

Anticonvulsants are used in the treatment of bipolar disorder as mood stabilizers. Originally developed for the treatment of epilepsy, they have been shown to relieve the symptoms of mania and reduce mood swings.

Valproic acid (Depakote®, Depakene®, Depakine®)

Valproic acid, also known as divalproex or valproate, is a highly effective mood stabilizer. Common brand names include Depakote® and Depakene®. Valproic acid is often the first choice for rapid cycling, mixed mania, or mania with hallucinations or delusions. It is a good bipolar medication option if lithium is not tolerated.

Common side effects include:

- Drowsiness
- Weight gain
- Dizziness
- Tremor
- Diarrhea
- Nausea

Carbamazepine (Tegretol®)

Carbamazepine is used off-label as a second-line treatment for bipolar disorder and in combination with an antipsychotic in some cases of schizophrenia when treatment with a conventional antipsychotic alone has failed. The drug may also be effective for ADHD.

Potential side effects include, among others, a rare aplastic anemia and agranulocytosis and more commonly, there are minor changes such as decreased white blood cell or platelet counts, that do not seem to progress to more serious problems. Increased risks of suicide, increased risks of hyponatremia and SIADH, risks to the fetus in women who are pregnant, specifically congenital malformations like spina bifida, and developmental disorders have also been reported.

Common adverse effects may include drowsiness, dizziness, headaches and migraines, motor coordination impairment, nausea, vomiting, and/or constipation. Alcohol use while taking carbamazepine may lead to enhanced depression of the central nervous system. Less common side effects may include increased risk of seizures in people with mixed seizure disorders, abnormal heart rhythms, blurry or double vision. Also, rare case reports of an auditory side effect have been made, whereby patients perceive sounds about a semitone lower than previously; this unusual side effect is usually not noticed by most people and disappears after the person stops taking carbamazepine.

Carbamazepine has a potential for drug interactions; caution should be used in combining other medicines with it, including other antiepileptics and mood stabilizers.

Having an eye on the liver function is advisable, especially in cases with preexisting liver conditions. Prospective studies indicate that a sizeable proportion of patients taking carbamazepine have transient serum aminotransferase elevations (ranging from 1% to 22%). These elevations are usually benign, not associated with liver histological abnormalities and usually resolve even with drug continuation. In addition, most patients on carbamazepine develop mild-to-moderate elevations in gamma glutamyltranspeptidase (GGT) levels, probably indicative of hepatic enzyme induction rather than liver injury. Marked aminotransferase elevations (more than 5-fold elevated) occur less frequently.

Lamotrigine (Lamictal®)

Lamotrigine is approved in the US for maintenance treatment of bipolar I disorder and bipolar II disorder. While the anticonvulsants carbamazepine and valproate are predominantly antimanics, lamotrigine is most effective for preventing the recurrent depressive episodes of bipolar disorder. The drug seems ineffective in the treatment of current rapid-cycling, acute mania, or acute depression in bipolar disorder; however, it is effective at prevention of or delaying of manic, depressive, or rapid cycling episodes. Lamotrigine may treat bipolar depression without triggering mania, hypomania, mixed states, or rapid-cycling.

It is frequently recommended in bipolar maintenance when depression is prominent and that more research is needed in regard to its role in the treatment of acute bipolar depression and unipolar depression. Furthermore, no information to recommend its use in other psychiatric disorders was found.

Lamotrigine prescribing information has a black box warning about life-threatening skin reactions, including Stevens–Johnson syndrome (SJS), DRESS syndrome and toxic epidermal necrolysis (TEN). Patients should seek medical attention for any unexpected skin rash immediately, as its presence is an indication of a possible serious or even deadly side-effect of the drug. Not all rashes that occur while taking lamotrigine progress to SJS or TEN. Between 5 and 10% of patients will develop a rash, but only one in a thousand patients will develop a serious rash. Rash and other skin reactions are more common in children, so this medication is often reserved for adults. For patients whose lamotrigine has been stopped after development of a rash, re-challenge with lamotrigine is also a viable option. However, it is not applicable for very serious cases.

There is also an increased incidence of these eruptions in patients who are currently on, or recently discontinued a valproate-type anticonvulsant drug, as these medications interact in such a way that the clearance of both is decreased and the effective dose of lamotrigine is increased.

Other side-effects include loss of balance or coordination; double vision; crossed eyes; pupil constriction; blurred vision; dizziness and lack of coordination; drowsiness, insomnia; anxiety; vivid dreams or nightmares; dry mouth, mouth ulcers; memory problems; mood changes; itchiness; runny nose; cough; nausea, indigestion, abdominal pain, weight loss; missed or painful menstrual periods; and vaginitis. The side-effect profile varies for different patient populations

Many studies have found no association between lamotrigine exposure in utero and birth defects, while those that have found an association have found only slight associations with minor malformations like cleft palates. Review studies have found that overall rates of congenital malformations in infants exposed to lamotrigine in utero are relatively low (1-4%), which is similar to the rate of malformations in the general population. Lamotrigine is expressed in breast milk, however

Antipsychotics

Antipsychotics been found to help with regular manic episodes, and they may be a second-line choice if the mood stabilizers mentioned above have failed. Often, antipsychotic medications are combined with a mood stabilizer such as lithium or valproic acid.

Second-generation antipsychotic medications used for bipolar disorder include:

    Olanzapine (Zyprexa®)
    Quetiapine (Seroquel®)
    Risperidone (Risperdal®)
    Aripiprazole (Abilify®)

Ziprasidone (Geodon®) is used more rarely.

Clozapine (Clozaril®) is used in cases where the other second-generation antipsychotic drugs do not work. However, because of a relatively rare but potentially lethal agranulocytosis, regular counts of white blood cells are required.

Common side effects of antipsychotic medications for bipolar disorder are

> Drowsiness
> Weight gain (particularly olanzapine)
> Sexual dysfunction
> Dry mouth
> Constipation
> Blurred vision

Sexual and erectile dysfunction is a common side effect of antipsychotic medications, one that often deters bipolar disorder patients from continuing medication. A recent study has shown that the medication Sildenafil citrate (Viagra®) is relatively effective in the treatment of antipsychotic-induced erectile dysfunction in men, but it may in many cases be better to switch the antipsychotic medication, which can make the problem disappear. Also, it needs to be remembered that it may sometimes be the underlying psychiatric condition that causes the sexual dysfunction.

All antipsychotics, with the apparent exception of Clozapine, can potentially cause late dyskinesia, which is in many cases untreatable. Some may also prolong the QT interval more than others, which makes an ECG part of good practice before administering a second-generation antipsychotic.

Other Substances

Benzodiazepines

Mood stabilizers can take up to several weeks to reach their full effect. In the meantime, benzodiazepines can bring some relief of anxiety, agitation, or insomnia. Benzodiazepines are fast-acting sedatives that work within 30 minutes to an hour. Because of their high addictive potential, however, benzodiazepines should only be used until the mood stabilizer or antidepressant begins to work. A history of substance abuse requires special caution.

Calcium channel blockers

Traditionally used to treat heart problems and high blood pressure, they also have a mood stabilizing effect. They have fewer side effects than traditional mood stabilizers, but they are also less effective. However, they may be an option for people who cannot tolerate lithium or anticonvulsants.

Thyroid hormone

People with bipolar disorder often have abnormal levels of thyroid hormone. Thyroid dysfunction is particularly prevalent in rapid cyclers. Lithium treatment can also cause low thyroid levels. In these cases, thyroid medication is added to the drug treatment regimen. While research is still ongoing, thyroid medication also shows promise as a treatment for bipolar depression with minimal side effects.

Antidepressants

Mounting evidence suggests that antidepressants are not effective in the treatment of bipolar depression. A major study funded by the National Institute of Mental Health showed that adding an antidepressant to a mood stabilizer was no more effective in treating bipolar depression than using a mood stabilizer alone. Another NIHM study found that antidepressants work no better than placebo. Antidepressants can trigger mania in people with bipolar disorder.

Mood stabilizer plus antidepressant

There may be cases where a mood stabilizer cannot be switched, and an antidepressant needs to be added to prevent the patient from falling into too extreme lows. If antidepressants are used at all, they should be combined with a mood stabilizer such as lithium or valproic acid. Taking an antidepressant without a mood stabilizer is likely to trigger a manic episode.

There are differences among antidepressants. Venlafaxine has been shown to be most likely to push a patient into a manic episode and Bupropion (Wellbutrin®) is probably least likely to cause a manic episode, with the SSRIs being somewhere in between. No antidepressant can be considered as 'safe' for the use in bipolar conditions, but it makes good sense to start with an antidepressant that is less likely to cause a manic episode. If the depression is severe, one may have to resort to an antidepressant which is more activating, but in most cases changing the mood stabilizer is the preferred option.

If antidepressants are discontinued, the tapering process may have to be done slowly to reduce adverse withdrawal effects. Venlafaxine (Effexor®) is an example. However, antidepressants may have to be stopped immediately if any symptoms of mania or hypomania develop.

Non-Pharmacological Approaches

Psychotherapy

In any case, it should be kept in mind that patients on medication for bipolar disorder tend to recover much faster and control their moods much better if they also get psychotherapy. Even if therapy sessions are at longer intervals, they can of great help to a patient suffering from a bipolar condition through a greater sense of safety, building greater self-confidence and supporting the patient in his or her daily life.

Exercise

Getting regular exercise can reduce bipolar disorder symptoms and help stabilize mood swings. Exercise is also a safe and effective way to release the pent-up energy associated with the manic episodes of bipolar disorder.

Sleep hygiene

Studies have found that insufficient sleep can precipitate manic episodes in bipolar patients. To keep symptoms and mood episodes to a minimum a stable sleep schedule should be maintained. It is also important to regulate darkness and light exposure as these throw off sleep-wake cycles and upset the sensitive biological clock in people with bipolar disorder.

Healthy diet

Weight gain is a common side effect of many bipolar medications, so it is important to adopt healthy eating habits. Caffeine, alcohol, and drugs should be avoided as they can adversely interact with bipolar medications. Omega-3 fatty acids may lessen the symptoms of bipolar disorder.

Social support network

Living with bipolar disorder can be challenging and having a solid support system in place can make all the difference in one's outlook and motivation. Participating in a bipolar disorder support group allows the sharing of experiences and learning from others. Support from loved ones also makes a huge difference.

Social Anxiety

Social anxiety should primarily be treated with psychotherapy. However, medication can be effective as a support. Reducing anxiety with the help of medication can make it easier for patients to train their skills in social settings. Some drugs work well in the short run, others are better and safer to use in the long-run. Often in the beginning a two-fold strategy is used to help people with their symptoms fast and then have a long-term strategy in place for lasting improvements.

Anxiolytics

Anxiolytics, particularly the benzodiazepines, often reduce the level of anxiety quite effectively and are the most widely prescribed medication to reduce anxiety sporadically. Although they often work quickly, they can be habit-forming and sedating, so they typically should be prescribed only for short-term use. They should also be tried before encountering an anxiety provoking social situation to get a sense for their effect. Also, they should not be combined with alcohol as this could lead to a potentiation of the sedative effect. Unfortunately, social situations often come with alcohol. They should also not be used if a lowering of inhibitions or critical reasoning can get one in unwanted or even dangerous situations, or while driving or operating heavy machinery. Still, having said all this, they can be valuable in the more severe kinds of social anxiety conditions to allow an affected individual to get involved in daily life again.

Lorazepam, Alprazolam and even Diazepam, can be effective in low doses, taken irregularly in the short-run, if combined with therapy and an SSRI, both of which can take a while to work. If the alternative is self-medication with alcohol, anything that supports the patient in a supervised fashion should be welcomed. However, this requires willingness and motivation on the side of the patient not to take the medication and consume alcohol concurrently.

The benzodiazepines can take up to 45 minutes to an hour to work, while a sublingual preparation of lorazepam acts quite fast, often within 15 minutes. The goal should be to enable patients to use their skills learned in therapy to tolerate and interact in social situations.

Selective serotonin reuptake inhibitors (SSRIs)

A more future oriented and over the long-run more effective treatment consists of selective serotonin reuptake inhibitors (SSRIs), antidepressants, which also help against anxiety and panic attacks. Since social anxiety is often linked to clinical or slightly subclinical anxiety or depression, they may be worth considering. Several types of antidepressants other than the SSRIs can theoretically be used to treat social anxiety disorder, including the serotonin-norepinephrine reuptake inhibitor (SNRI) Venlafaxine (Effexor® an others) and, to a lesser extent, the noradrenergic and specific serotonergic antidepressant (NaSSA) Mirtazapine (Remeron® and others). However, selective serotonin reuptake inhibitors (SSRIs) are often the first type of medication tried for persistent symptoms of social anxiety. The reasons are mostly empirical and anecdotal as they seem to work in practice, while having a relatively benign profile of possible side-effects. Venlafaxine may increase anxiety and panic attacks in the early phase of treatment.

The SSRIs increase level of the neurotransmitter serotonin in the synaptic cleft between the endings of nerve fibers from (mostly different) nerve cells. This leads to a change in the receptor density of certain serotonin receptor subclasses in the cell membrane and thereby directly reflects the flow of information between and through nerve cells. The SSRIs are effective against anxiety of all kinds, including obsessive-compulsive disorder, and depression. Especially after they came out, they received bad press that they change one's personality and lead to addiction. However, the current consensus is that they do not radically change one's personality and they are generally thought as being non-addictive. There is some concern over an emotional flattening in the long-run, but this has not been convincingly demonstrated yet. In clinical experience, they still represent a relatively favorable tradeoff between the more common side-effects and the change in the quality of life they can bring about. Discontinuing them is quite simple, but still should be discussed and the pros and cons weighed off carefully, not just if suicidality is an issue. The old symptoms may resurface after discontinuation, especially if they have been taken for less than a year. Recommendations vary for anxiety and depression, but there seems to be a consensus that they should be taken for a longer period if the clinical diagnosis justifies it.

It may take several weeks to several months of treatment for the clinical symptoms to noticeably improve. The reason why antidepressant medication affecting the serotonin system may take longer is because the number of receptors (density) in the cell membrane, which translate chemical signals into other chemical signals, but more importantly into fast moving electric signals along the cell membrane, must be changed. This requires transcription and translation from the DNA code into some receptor proteins and the 'recycling' of others.

Other Options

Among the other options are the following:

Beta blockers

These substances block the stimulating effect of epinephrine (adrenaline). They may reduce heart rate, blood pressure, pounding of the heart, and shaking voice and limbs. Because of that, they may work best when used infrequently to control symptoms for a particular situation, such as giving a speech. They're not recommended for general treatment of social anxiety disorder. They should be tried out before encountering an anxiety provoking situations to psychologically decrease the anxiety of experiencing anxiety during the event.

Beta blockers are the only medication that tends to be used more often with social anxiety than other anxiety disorders. These are drugs like Propranolol that prevent the body from experiencing any profound anxiety symptoms. How they work is not entirely known, but it is believed that they prevent the heart from getting excited, which keeps the body calm in anxiety situations.

Buspirone

Buspirone (Buspar®) is a mild anxiolytic with few side effects, which is generally well tolerated. The main problem with buspirone is that the effect is often too weak.

There are a few other social anxiety medications, but those mentioned above four are the most common. In the past, other drugs like MAO inhibitors were used, but they have since fallen out of favor because of their unfavorable side-effect profiles.

Psychotherapy

In any case, it is important to keep in mind that in the long-run the emphasis for social anxiety should be on psychotherapy rather than medication. There is probably a beneficial effect of medication if taken over the long-run as the brain learns to be less anxious and less worried about experiencing anxiety in social situations. However, this effect is likely to wear off if working on the underlying issues is avoided.

Schizophrenia

Schizophrenia in virtually all cases requires lifelong treatment, even when symptoms have subsided. Treatment includes better coping skills in everyday life, strategies to reduce stress and become aware of early warning signs of a psychotic episode, psychotherapy to better manage life, and medication. Medication may be life-long but does not have to be.

Schizophrenia affects a person's perception of the reality shared with other people. It can thus affect many areas in life, a patient's interaction with others, the workplace and relationships. Medication can help the patient reintegrate into society and interact in more meaningful ways.

Medication for an independent, autonomous life

Treatment with medication (antipsychotics) and psychosocial therapy can help manage the condition. In some cases, hospitalization may be needed. However, medication has drastically reduced the need for hospitalization or at least reduced the length per hospital stay. Many patients who had to be hospitalized for most of their lives in earlier times can now care for their families, work as highly paid managers in large corporations or be successful artists.

Medication allows people with schizophrenia to lead normal lives. Especially the newer generation of antipsychotics has increased the quality of life significantly, while reducing some of the side-effects of the earlier generation of antipsychotic medication. Still, antipsychotic medication has overall still not reached the low side-effect profiles of newer antidepressants. While tardive dyskinesia has become rarer with the second-generation antipsychotics (SGAs) and is virtually absent in clozapine especially and the potentially lethal malignant neuroleptic syndrome is a very rare phenomenon, they are often associated with side-effects from weight gain (especially olanzapine) to drowsiness (quetiapine). It seems that we are only willing to accept the greater potential side-effects of modern antipsychotics because of the enormous improvement they can bring in a patient's quality of life.

Psychotherapy should be added in the beginning and for low-frequency follow-up. Everyone benefits from a less stressful life which is more in sync with one's values and interests, but especially do individuals with a diagnosis of schizophrenia, or any other psychotic, anxiety, mood or personality disorder. This often means working with the past and the future in the present for a more integrative, complete effect.

The dopamine hypothesis

Medication still is the cornerstone of schizophrenia treatment. Antipsychotic drugs are thought to control symptoms by affecting the dopamine neurotransmission system in the brain. It may not be the effect that directly brings about relief from psychotic symptoms, but all drugs used at present in the treatment of schizophrenia have an affinity for the dopamine system, some almost exclusively, some in combination with other neurotransmitter systems.

Dopamine D2 and D4 receptors

Blocking or partially blocking the effect of dopamine at the D2 and D4 receptors in the synapses between nerve fibers (and also outside the synapses) seems to be effective against the positive symptoms of schizophrenia, such as hallucinations and paranoia. This is called the dopamine hypothesis. Much empirical evidence supports the hypothesis that there is too much or too little dopamine activity in various centers of the brain in patients suffering from schizophrenia.

Other Neurotransmitter Systems

There are interactions between the dopamine system and other neurotransmitter systems, such as the serotonin neurotransmission, and it is unclear which system and area of the brain plays the decisive role in the onset and maintenance of schizophrenia and related psychotic disorders. Also, antipsychotic drugs usually have an effect on multiple neurotransmitter systems, and it still not entirely clear how they interact with each other to increase or decrease therapeutic and side effects.

Receptor affinity, effectiveness and side-effects

The complex effect of antipsychotics in various centers of the brain and the effect of antipsychotics on various neurotransmitter systems and various receptor subclasses is responsible for the variety of effects and side-effects of an antipsychotic.

Some 'side-effects' might be desirable. Newer antipsychotics with an effect on the serotonin transmitter pathway, such as Olanzapine (Zyprexa®), may, for example, be useful in some cases of sleep abnormalities, eating disorders and obsessive thoughts. The fact that Olanzapine (Zyprexa®) has a sedative effect is preferred by many patients to help them sleep. In some cases, it is used as a non-addictive sleep medication, although sleep inducing antidepressants are here to be preferred because of the usually better side-effect profile.

Monotreatment and lowest effective dose

The goal of treatment with antipsychotic medications is to effectively manage signs and symptoms at the lowest possible dose. Unfortunately, minimum effective doses have not been studied as extensively as the side-effects. The preference should always be for the use of a single substance (monotreatment), but in some cases, this may not be possible. Switching the antipsychotic, especially from the second generation, in many cases allows for monotreatment with one substance.

Compliance

Because medications for schizophrenia can cause serious side effects, people with schizophrenia may be reluctant to take them. Willingness to cooperate with treatment may affect drug choice. For example, someone who is likely to forget medication in the sense of being ambivalent towards it, especially in psychotic phases, may need to be given injections instead of taking a pill. Among the most serious side-effects are the extrapyramidal symptoms (EPS) including tardive dyskinesia, a condition with involuntary movements which is largely untreatable. But antipsychotics can also have an effect the functioning of the heart (QT prolongation), blood cells and enzymes, the liver and other organs.

First-generation antipsychotics

The first-generation antipsychotics have frequent and potentially significant neurological side effects, including the possibility of developing a movement disorder (tardive dyskinesia) that may or may not be reversible. First-generation antipsychotics include:

> Chlorpromazine
> Fluphenazine
> Haloperidol (Haldol®)
> Perphenazine

These antipsychotics are often cheaper than second-generation antipsychotics, especially the generic versions, which can be a consideration when long-term treatment is necessary, but the better side-effect profile of the second-generation antipsychotics should outweigh this. Especially in psychiatric emergencies or when second-generation antipsychotics are not effective enough drugs like Haloperidol may have to be used, still with the aim to replace it with a second-generation antipsychotic in the future. However, in some cases an acceptable quality of life cannot be obtained without the use of the old first-generation antipsychotics.

Second-generation antipsychotics

These newer, second-generation medications are generally preferred because they pose a lower risk of serious side effects than do first-generation antipsychotics. The most important representatives of the second-generation antipsychotics are:

> Aripiprazole (Abilify®)
> Olanzapine (Zyprexa®)
> Quetiapine (Seroquel®)
> Risperidone (Risperdal®)
>> and its active metabolite Paliperidone (Invega®)

Clozapine (Clozaril®) may be the only antipsychotic without the risk of EPS. However, it can cause the rare, but potentially lethal condition of agranulocytosis.

Trauma

Disconnection

Trauma leads to a disconnect from oneself and the world. Medication should not increase the various forms of dissociation patients often experience but create a healthy distance to any feelings that might be overwhelming to the person and depleting his or her psychological resources. This also helps the patient to get the most from a concurrent psychotherapy and focus on daily living, tasks and challenges, which can have a stabilizing effect.

Psychotherapy and Medication

The treatment of trauma primarily requires psychotherapy, while medication can support and facilitate the process. Medication can play an important role in reducing the symptoms to a level which allows the reintegration of an individual into society, a more positive sense of the future and frequently facilitates psychotherapy by improving communication between the patient and his or her environment.

Second Generation Antipsychotics

If there are dissociative symptoms, neuroleptics can be useful in re-establishing an integrated sense of the person and a healthy core sense of self. Atypical (or second generation) neuroleptics should be used, if possible, although they too can have various potential side-effects and contraindications which need to be kept in mind. Only in the most extreme cases should one have to resort to clozapine, and just in the rarest of cases to one of the older typical neuroleptics, such as haloperidol. Much depends on the severity of symptoms and the patient's attitude towards medication.

Selective Serotonin Reuptake Inhibitors (SSRIs)

Flashbacks and hypersensitivity to one's own emotions and those of others can often be dealt with effectively using an antidepressant from the group of SSRIs, while older tricyclics can be of help as well, especially if extra sedation is desired. However, victims of severe traumata can also be suicidal which makes the SSRIs a safer choicer.

Benzodiazepines

Benzodiazepines as an add on can be useful, if there is a high level of anxiety or agitation and restlessness. However, the antidepressants and/or neuroleptics should make their use sporadic. Also, any suicidal tendencies should be kept in mind when they are prescribed and the possible paradoxical effect in patients with some forms of personality disorder and trauma. In the latter, benzodiazepines can increase the sense of void and emptiness, and thus the risk of suicidality.

Supportive to Daily Living and Psychotherapy

Generally, medication should always be supportive to patients in their daily lives and to the psychotherapeutic process. This means that patients should not be so sedated that they are unable to feel themselves. At the same time, they should feel distanced enough from painful emotions, so as not to feel overwhelmed when they are addressed constructively in therapy.

Attention Deficit Hyperactivity Disorder (ADHD)

Stimulants are frequently used to treat attention deficit-hyperactivity disorder. A stimulant is a drug that stimulates the central nervous system, increasing arousal, attention and endurance. Because the medications can be addictive, patients with a history of drug abuse are typically monitored closely or treated with a non-stimulant. It is argued that the risk of addiction in patients diagnosed with ADHD is much lower.

There are also some antidepressants that have stimulant effects.

Common stimulants include:

> **Methylphenidate** (Ritalin®, Concerta®), a norepinephrine-dopamine reuptake inhibitor
> **Dextroamphetamine** (Dexedrine®), the dextro-enantiomer of amphetamine
> **Dexmethylphenidate** (Focalin®), the active dextro-enantiomer of methylphenidate
> **Lisdexamfetamine** (Vyvanse®), a prodrug containing the dextro-enantiomer of amphetamine
> There are also mixed amphetamine salts, such as Adderall®, a 3:1 mix of dextro/levo-enantiomers of amphetamine.

Methylphenidate

Methylphenidate hydrochloride USP is a mild central nervous system (CNS) stimulant, available in immediate or long-acting preparations. It presumably activates the brain stem arousal system and cortex to produce its stimulant effect.

Effects on the QT interval

In one study, the maximum mean prolongation of QTcF intervals was <5 ms, and the upper limit of the 90% confidence interval was below 10 ms for all time matched comparisons versus placebo. This was below the threshold of clinical concern and there was no evident-exposure response relationship.

Ritalin is indicated as an integral part of a total treatment program which typically includes other remedial measures (psychological, educational, social) for a stabilizing effect in children with a behavioral syndrome characterized by the following group of developmentally inappropriate symptoms: moderate-to-severe distractibility, short attention span, hyperactivity, emotional lability, and impulsivity. The diagnosis of this syndrome should not be made with finality when these symptoms are only of comparatively recent origin. Non-localizing neurological signs, learning disability, and abnormal EEG may or may not be present, and a diagnosis of central nervous system dysfunction may or may not be warranted.

Drug treatment is not indicated for all children with this syndrome. Stimulants are not intended for use in the child who exhibits symptoms secondary to environmental factors and/or primary psychiatric disorders, including psychosis. Appropriate educational placement is essential and psychosocial intervention is generally necessary. When remedial measures alone are insufficient, the decision to prescribe stimulant medication will depend upon the physician's assessment of the chronicity and severity of the child's symptoms.

Contraindications

Marked anxiety, tension, and agitation are contraindications to Ritalin, since the drug may aggravate these symptoms. Ritalin is contraindicated also in patients known to be hypersensitive to the drug, in patients with glaucoma, and in patients with motor tics or with a family history or diagnosis of Tourette's syndrome.

Ritalin is contraindicated during treatment with monoamine oxidase inhibitors, and within a minimum of 14 days following discontinuation of a monoamine oxidase inhibitor (hypertensive crises may result).

Hypertension and Other Cardiovascular Conditions

Stimulant medications cause a modest increase in average blood pressure (about 2-4 mmHg) and average heart rate (about 3-6 bpm), and individuals may have larger increases. While the mean changes alone would not be expected to have short-term consequences, all patients should be monitored for larger changes in heart rate and blood pressure. Caution is indicated in treating patients whose underlying medical conditions might be compromised by increases in blood pressure or heart rate, e.g., those with preexisting hypertension, heart failure, recent myocardial infarction, or ventricular arrhythmia.

Assessing Cardiovascular Status in Patients being Treated with Stimulant Medications

Children, adolescents, or adults who are being considered for treatment with stimulant medications should have a careful history (including assessment for a family history of sudden death or ventricular arrhythmia) and physical exam to assess for the presence of cardiac disease and should receive further cardiac evaluation if findings suggest such disease (e.g., electrocardiogram and echocardiogram). Patients who develop symptoms such as exertional chest pain, unexplained syncope, or other symptoms suggestive of cardiac disease during stimulant treatment should undergo a prompt cardiac evaluation.

Serious Cardiovascular Events

Children and Adolescents

Sudden death has been reported in association with CNS stimulant treatment at usual doses in children and adolescents with structural cardiac abnormalities or other serious heart problems. Although some serious heart problems alone carry an increased risk of sudden death, stimulant products generally should not be used in children or adolescents with known serious structural cardiac abnormalities, cardiomyopathy, serious heart rhythm abnormalities, or other serious cardiac problems that may place them at increased vulnerability to the sympathomimetic effects of a stimulant drug.

Adults

Sudden death, stroke, and myocardial infarction have been reported in adults taking stimulant drugs at usual doses for ADHD. Although the role of stimulants in these adult cases is also unknown, adults have a greater likelihood than children of having serious structural cardiac abnormalities, cardiomyopathy, serious heart rhythm abnormalities, coronary artery disease, or other serious cardiac problems. Adults with such abnormalities should also generally not be treated with stimulant drugs.

Psychiatric Adverse Events

Preexisting Psychosis

Administration of stimulants may exacerbate symptoms of behavior disturbance and thought disorder in patients with a preexisting psychotic disorder.

Bipolar Disorder

Particular care should be taken in using stimulants to treat ADHD in patients with comorbid bipolar disorder because of concern for possible induction of a mixed/ manic episode in such patients. Prior to initiating treatment with a stimulant, patients with comorbid depressive symptoms should be adequately screened to determine if they are at risk for bipolar disorder; such screening should include a detailed psychiatric history, including a family history of suicide, bipolar disorder, and depression.

Emergence of New Psychotic or Manic Symptoms

Treatment emergent psychotic or manic symptoms, e. g., hallucinations, delusional thinking, or mania in children and adolescents without a prior history of psychotic illness or mania can be caused by stimulants at usual doses. If such symptoms occur, consideration should be given to a possible causal role of the stimulant, and discontinuation of treatment may be appropriate. In a pooled analysis of multiple short-term, placebo-controlled studies, such symptoms occurred in about 0.1% (4 patients with events out of 3,482 exposed to methylphenidate or amphetamine for several weeks at usual doses) of stimulant-treated patients compared to 0 in placebo-treated patients.

Aggression

Aggressive behavior or hostility is often observed in children and adolescents with ADHD and has been reported in clinical trials and the post-marketing experience of some medications indicated for the treatment of ADHD. Although there is no systematic evidence that stimulants cause aggressive behavior or hostility, patients beginning treatment for ADHD should be monitored for the appearance of or worsening of aggressive behavior or hostility.

Long-Term Suppression of Growth

Careful follow-up of weight and height in children ages 7 to 10 years who were randomized to either methylphenidate or non-medication treatment groups over 14 months, as well as in naturalistic subgroups of newly methylphenidate-treated and non-medication treated children over 36 months (to the ages of 10 to 13 years), suggests that consistently medicated children (i.e., treatment for 7 days per week throughout the year) have a temporary slowing in growth rate (on average, a total of about 2 cm less growth in height and 2.7 kg less growth in weight over 3 years), without evidence of growth rebound during this period of development. Published data are inadequate to determine whether chronic use of amphetamines may cause a similar suppression of growth, however, it is anticipated that they likely have this effect as well. Therefore, growth should be monitored during treatment with stimulants, and patients who are not growing or gaining height or weight as expected may need to have their treatment interrupted.

Seizures

There is some clinical evidence that stimulants may lower the convulsive threshold in patients with prior history of seizures, in patients with prior EEG abnormalities in absence of seizures, and, very rarely, in patients without a history of seizures and no prior EEG evidence of seizures. In the presence of seizures, the drug should be discontinued.

Priapism

Prolonged and painful erections, sometimes requiring surgical intervention, have been reported with methylphenidate products in both pediatric and adult patients. Priapism was not reported with drug initiation but developed after some time on the drug, often subsequent to an increase in dose. Priapism has also appeared during a period of drug withdrawal (drug holidays or during discontinuation). Patients who develop abnormally sustained or frequent and painful erections should seek immediate medical attention.

Peripheral Vasculopathy, Including Raynaud's Phenomenon

Stimulants, including Ritalin and Ritalin-SR, used to treat ADHD are associated with peripheral vasculopathy, including Raynaud's phenomenon. Signs and symptoms are usually intermittent and mild; however, very rare sequelae include digital ulceration and/or soft tissue breakdown. Effects of peripheral vasculopathy, including Raynaud's phenomenon, were observed in post-marketing reports at different times and at therapeutic doses in all age groups throughout the course of treatment. Signs and symptoms generally improve after reduction in dose or discontinuation of drug. Careful observation for digital changes is necessary during treatment with ADHD stimulants. Further clinical evaluation (e.g., rheumatology referral) may be appropriate for certain patients.

Visual Disturbance

Difficulties with accommodation and blurring of vision have been reported with stimulant treatment.

Use in Children Under Six Years of Age

Ritalin should not be used in children under 6 years, since safety and efficacy in this age group have not been established.

Drug Dependence

Ritalin should be given cautiously to patients with a history of drug dependence or alcoholism. Chronic abusive use can lead to marked tolerance and psychological dependence with varying degrees of abnormal behavior. Frank psychotic episodes can occur, especially with parenteral abuse. Careful supervision is required during withdrawal from abusive use, since severe depression may occur. Withdrawal following chronic therapeutic use may unmask symptoms of the underlying disorder that may require follow-up.

Drug Interactions

Ritalin should not be used in patients being treated (currently or within the proceeding two weeks) with MAO Inhibitors (see CONTRAINDICATIONS, Monoamine Oxidase Inhibitors). Because of possible effects on blood pressure, Ritalin should be used cautiously with pressor agents.

Methylphenidate may decrease the effectiveness of drugs used to treat hypertension. Methylphenidate is metabolized primarily to Ritalinic acid by de-esterification and not through oxidative pathways.

Human pharmacologic studies have shown that racemic methylphenidate may inhibit the metabolism of coumarin anticoagulants, anticonvulsants (e.g., phenobarbital, phenytoin, primidone), and tricyclic drugs (e.g., imipramine, clomipramine, desipramine). Downward dose adjustments of these drugs may be required when given concomitantly with methylphenidate. It may be necessary to adjust the dosage and monitor plasma drug concentration (or, in case of coumarin, coagulation times), when initiating or discontinuing methylphenidate.

Carcinogenesis/Mutagenesis

In a lifetime carcinogenicity study carried out in B6C3F1 mice, methylphenidate caused an increase in hepatocellular adenomas and, in males only, an increase in hepatoblastomas, at a daily dose of approximately 60 mg/kg/day. This dose is approximately 30 times and 4 times the maximum recommended human dose on a mg/kg and mg/m2 basis, respectively. Hepatoblastoma is a relatively rare rodent malignant tumor type. There was no increase in total malignant hepatic tumors. The mouse strain used is sensitive to the development of hepatic tumors, and the significance of these results to humans is unknown.

Methylphenidate did not cause any increases in tumors in a lifetime carcinogenicity study carried out in F344 rats; the highest dose used was approximately 45 mg/kg/day, which is approximately 22 times and 5 times the maximum recommended human dose on a mg/kg and mg/m2 basis, respectively.

In a 24-week carcinogenicity study in the transgenic mouse strain p53+/-, which is sensitive to genotoxic carcinogens, there was no evidence of carcinogenicity. Male and female mice were fed diets containing the same concentration of methylphenidate as in the lifetime carcinogenicity study; the high-dose groups were exposed to 60-74 mg/kg/day of methylphenidate.

Methylphenidate was not mutagenic in the in vitro Ames reverse mutation assay or in the in vitro mouse lymphoma cell forward mutation assay. Sister chromatid exchanges and chromosome aberrations were increased, indicative of a weak clastogenic response, in an in vitro assay in cultured Chinese Hamster Ovary (CHO) cells. Methylphenidate was negative in vivo in males and females in the mouse bone marrow micronucleus assay.

Impairment of Fertility

Methylphenidate did not impair fertility in male or female mice that were fed diets containing the drug in an 18-week Continuous Breeding study. The study was conducted at doses up to 160 mg/kg/day, approximately 80-fold and 8-fold the highest recommended dose on a mg/kg and mg/m2 basis, respectively.

Pregnancy

Pregnancy Category C

Adverse Reactions

Nervousness and insomnia are the most common adverse reactions but are usually controlled by reducing dosage and omitting the drug in the afternoon or evening. Other reactions include hypersensitivity (including skin rash, urticaria, fever, arthralgia, exfoliative dermatitis, erythema multiforme with histopathological findings of necrotizing vasculitis, and thrombocytopenic purpura); anorexia; nausea; dizziness; palpitations; headache; dyskinesia; drowsiness; blood pressure and pulse changes, both up and down; tachycardia; angina; cardiac arrhythmia; abdominal pain; weight loss during prolonged therapy; libido changes. There have been rare reports of Tourette's syndrome. Toxic psychosis has been reported. Although a definite causal relationship has not been established, the following have been reported in patients taking this drug: serotonin syndrome in combination with serotonergic drugs, rhabdomyolysis, instances of abnormal liver function, ranging from transaminase elevation to severe hepatic injury; isolated cases of cerebral arteritis and/or occlusion; leukopenia and/or anemia; transient depressed mood; aggressive behavior; a few instances of scalp hair loss. Very rare reports of neuroleptic malignant syndrome (NMS) have been received, and, in most of these, patients were concurrently receiving therapies associated with NMS. In a single report, a 10-year-old boy who had been taking methylphenidate for approximately 18 months experienced an NMS-like event within 45 minutes of ingesting his first dose of venlafaxine. It is uncertain whether this case represented a drug-drug interaction, a response to either drug alone, or some other cause.

In children, loss of appetite, abdominal pain, weight loss during prolonged therapy, insomnia, and tachycardia may occur more frequently; however, any of the other adverse reactions listed above may also occur.

Tourette's

Clinically, significant improvements in Tourette's Syndrome on the pharmaceutical side can be accomplished with neuroleptics, which have an effect in the dopamine transmission system, which is thought to play a leading role in the symptoms of Tourette's Syndrome. Substances with a predominant inhibitory effect on the neural pathways that rely on the neurotransmitter dopamine are largely the neuroleptics or antipsychotics, so called because they are effective in the treatment of psychosis, such as schizophrenia. Olanzapine is frequently used. However, the potentially more serious side effects of the neuroleptics, even the second-generation antipsychotics, should be kept in mind. Weight can be a problem, particularly in the case of olanzapine.

Stress and anxiety can make Tourette's worse, which also points to a role for the serotonin transmission system, which plays a role in anxiety and depression. Thus, if anxiety seems to be a large factor in maintaining the Tourette's, an SSRI, such as escitalopram, may be helpful as an alternative. Also, if neuroleptics alone do not yield the desired effect, adding on an SSRI can increase the effectiveness of the neuroleptic. However, whenever combining an antidepressant with a neuroleptic, possible cross interactions should be kept in mind. Several neuroleptics affect the serotonin system, which can then in combination with an SSRI at least in theory lead to a potentially fatal serotonin syndrome.

In the long-term, psychotherapy can deliver good results if sources of stress and anxiety are identified and strategies developed to deal with them more effectively.

Weight Gain and the Metabolic Syndrome

People with severe mental illness, including schizophrenia and related psychotic disorders, bipolar disorder and major depressive disorder (MDD), experience a two-three times higher mortality rate than the general population (1, 2). The mortality gap translates into a 10-20 year shortened life expectancy (3, 4) and appears to be widening (5).

About 60% of the excess mortality observed in patients with severe mental illness (SMI) is due to physical comorbidities, predominantly cardiovascular diseases (6). Factors predisposing people with SMI to these conditions include

- antipsychotic medication and unhealthy lifestyles (7) and
- the lower probability to receive standard levels of medical care (8-12).

Metabolic Syndrome

Meta-analyses (13-16) documented that people with severe mental illness have an increased risk for developing metabolic syndrome compared with the general population.

Patients with schizophrenia and bipolar disorder seem to be at similar risk of developing it. (17) The prevalence appears higher in individuals with multi-episode schizophrenia compared with persons in their first episode. 14,18[22, 35] The relative metabolic syndrome risk compared to the general population is greatest in younger people with SMI and those treated with antipsychotics 19,20[37, 38].

Metabolic syndrome is defined by a combination of

>   central obesity
>   high blood pressure
>   low high-density lipoprotein (HDL) cholesterol
>   elevated triglycerides and
>   hyperglycemia.

In the general population, these clustered risk factors have been associated with the development of cardiovascular disease and excess mortality (21-23).

Populations

Gender

Population studies showed no significant difference between men and women. (24,25).

Age

Increasing age appears a key predictor of metabolic syndrome in the general population and in people with severe mental illness. (15,26).

Antipsychotics

Antipsychotic medications is increasingly used as frontline treatments for bipolar disorder (27), major depressive disorder (28), anxiety and some personality disorders (particularly borderline personality disorder), next to its conventional use in treating psychosis. Studies suggest that all antipsychotic medications places patients at a higher risk for the metabolic syndrome than the general population. It appears that (11,29-32).

- the risk of metabolic syndrome is significantly higher with clozapine, followed by olanzapine.
- the risk of metabolic syndrome is significantly lower with aripiprazole than for other antipsychotics, including typical antipsychotics
- the risk of metabolic syndrome is not appreciably higher with amisulpride than it is for aripiprazole.

The lowest metabolic syndrome prevalence for aripiprazole is noteworthy, as antipsychotics with lower cardiometabolic risk profiles in short-term studies are often prescribed for higher risk patients in clinical care, which may lead to an even higher cardiometabolic risk for the other drugs (33).

Antidepressants

Several antidepressants from the group of serotonin reuptake inhibitors, the tricyclic antidepressants and mirtazapine, which has noradrenergic and serotonergic effects, and others have been linked to weight gain and the metabolic syndrome.

Studies found that some antidepressants may, in some circumstances, reduce hyperglycemia, normalize glucose homeostasis and increase insulin sensitivity, (34) whereas others, including tricyclic antidepressants, may exacerbate glycemic dysfunction or have little effect on glucose homeostasis (35,36).

Patients with atypical depression appear to have significantly higher levels of inflammatory markers, body mass index, waist circumference and triglycerides, and lower HDL cholesterol than those with melancholic depression (37).

Minimizing the Risk

People with severe mental illness are more likely than the general population to have unhealthy lifestyle behaviors which can increase the risk of metabolic syndrome and cardiovascular disease. They tend to be more likely to be sedentary (38), smoking (39) and having diets that are high in saturated fats and refined sugars, while low in fruit and vegetables (40).. Thus, screening for and trying to minimize risk factors should be a key priority in the multidisciplinary treatment of people with severe mental illness (41-44).

References

1. Osborn DPJ, Levy G, Nazareth I et al. Relative risk of cardiovascular and cancer mortality in people with severe

mental illness from the United Kingdom's General Practice Research Database. Arch Gen Psychiatry 2007;64:242-49.

2. Reininghaus U, Dutta R, Dazzan P et al. Mortality in schizophrenia and other psychoses: a 10-year follow-up of the ÆSOP first-episode cohort. Schizophr Bull 2015;41:664-73.

3. Chang CK, Hayes RD, Perera G et al. Life expectancy at birth for people with serious mental illness from a secondary mental health care case register in London, UK. PLoS One 2011;6:e19590.

4. Lawrence D, Hancock KJ, Kisely S. The gap in life expectancy from preventable physical illness in psychiatric patients in Western Australia: retrospective analysis of population based registers. BMJ 2013;346:f2539.

5. Saha S, Chant D, McGrath J. A systematic review of mortality in schizophrenia. Arch Gen Psychiatry 2007;64:1123-31.

6. Hoang U, Goldacre MJ, Stewart R. Avoidable mortality in people with schizophrenia or bipolar disorder in England. Acta Psychiatr Scand 2013;127:195-201.

7. De Hert M, Correll CU, Bobes J et al. Physical illness in patients with severe mental disorders. I. Prevalence, impact of medications and disparities in health care. World Psychiatry 2011;10:52-77.

8. Mitchell AJ, Lord O. Do deficits in cardiac care influence high mortality rates in schizophrenia? A systematic review and pooled analysis. J Psychopharmacol 2010;24(Suppl. 4):69-80.

9. Mitchell AJ, Lord O, Malone D. Differences in the prescribing of medication for physical disorders in individuals with v. without mental illness: meta-analysis. Br J Psychiatry 2012;201:435-43.

10. Mitchell AJ, Malone D, Doebbeling CC. Quality of medical care for people with and without comorbid mental illness and substance misuse: systematic review of comparative studies. Br J Psychiatry 2009;194:491-9.

11. De Hert M, Vancampfort D, Correll CU et al. Guidelines for screening and monitoring of cardiometabolic risk in schizophrenia: systematic evaluation. Br J Psychiatry 2011;199:99-105.

12. Mitchell AJ, Vancampfort D, Sweers K et al. Prevalence of metabolic syndrome and metabolic abnormalities in schizophrenia and related disorders – a systematic review and meta-analysis. Schizophr Bull 2013;39:306-18.

14. Mitchell AJ, Vancampfort D, De Herdt A et al. Is the prevalence of metabolic syndrome and metabolic abnormalities increased in early schizophrenia? A comparative meta-analysis of first episode, untreated and treated patients. Schizophr Bull 2013;39:295-305.

15. Vancampfort D, Vansteelandt K, Correll CU et al. Metabolic syndrome and metabolic abnormalities in bipolar disorder: a meta-analysis of prevalence rates and moderators. Am J Psychiatry 2013;170:265-74.

16. Vancampfort D, Correll CU, Wampers M et al. Metabolic syndrome and metabolic abnormalities in patients with

depression: a meta-analysis of prevalence rates and moderators. Psychol Med 2014;94:2017-28.

17. Bartoli F, Carrà G, Crocamo C et al. Bipolar disorder, schizophrenia, and metabolic syndrome. Am J Psychiatry 2013;170:927-8.

18. Vancampfort D, Wampers M, Mitchell AJ et al. A meta-analysis of cardio-metabolic abnormalities in drug naïve, first-episode and multi-episode patients with schizophrenia versus general population controls. World Psychiatry 2013;12:240-50.

19. De Hert M, van Winkel R, Van Eyck D et al. Prevalence of diabetes, metabolic syndrome and metabolic abnormalities in schizophrenia over the course of the illness: a cross-sectional study. Clin Pract Epidemiol Ment Health 2006;2:14.

20. De Hert M, Detraux J, van Winkel R et al. Metabolic and cardiovascular adverse effects associated with antipsychotic drugs. Nat Rev Endocrinol 2011;8:114-26.

21. Gami AS, Witt BJ, Howard DE et al. Metabolic syndrome and risk of incident cardiovascular events and death: a systematic review and meta-analysis of longitudinal studies. J Am Coll Cardiol 2007;49:403-14.

22. Galassi A, Reynolds K, He J. Metabolic syndrome and risk of cardiovascular disease: a meta-analysis. Am J Med 2006;119:812-9.

23. Mottillo S, Filion KB, Genest J et al. The metabolic syndrome and cardiovascular risk: a systematic review and meta-analysis. J Am Coll Cardiol 2010;56:1113-32.

24. Ford ES, Giles WH, Dietz WH. Prevalence of the metabolic syndrome among US adults: findings from the third National Health and Nutrition Examination Survey. JAMA 2002;287:356-9.

25. Park YW, Zhu S, Palaniappan L et al. The metabolic syndrome: prevalence and associated risk factor findings in the US population from the Third National Health and Nutrition Examination Survey, 1988-1994. Arch Intern Med 2003;163:427-36.

26. North BJ, Sinclair DA. The intersection between aging and cardiovascular disease. Circ Res 2012;110:1097-108.

27. Pillarella J, Higashi A, Alexander GC et al. Trends in use of second-generation antipsychotics for treatment of bipolar disorder in the United States, 1998-2009. Psychiatr Serv 2012;63:83-6.

28. Davidson JR. Major depressive disorder treatment guidelines in America and Europe. J Clin Psychiatry 2010;71:e04.

29. Duvall S, Tweedie R. A non-parametric 'trim and fill' method for assessing publication bias in meta-analysis. J Am Stat Assoc 2000;95:89-98.

30. Hammerman A, Dreiher J, Klang SH et al. Antipsychotics and diabetes: an age-related association. Ann Pharmacother 2008;42:1316-22.

31. Nielsen J, Skadhede S, Correll CU. Antipsychotics associated with the development of type 2 diabetes in antipsychotic-naïve schizophrenia patients. Neuropsychopharmacology 2010;35:1997-2004.

32. Correll CU, Robinson DG, Schooler NR et al. Cardiometabolic risk in first episode schizophrenia-spectrum disorder patients: baseline results from the RAISE-ETP Study. JAMA Psychiatry 2014;71:1350-63.

33. Kessing LV, Thomsen AF, Mogensen UB et al. Treatment with antipsychotics and the risk of diabetes in clinical practice. Br J Psychiatry 2010;197:266-71.

34. Hennings JM, Schaaf L, Fulda S. Glucose metabolism and antidepressant medication. Curr Pharm Des 2012;18:5900-19.

35. Mojtabai R. Antidepressant use and glycemic control. Psychopharmacology 2013;227:467-77.

36. Correl CU, Detraux J, De Lepeleire J et al. Effects of antipsychotics, antidepressants and mood stabilizers on risk for physical diseases in patients with schizophrenia, depression and bipolar disorder. World Psychiatry 2015;14:119-36.

37. Lamers F, Vogelzangs N, Merikangas KR et al. Evidence for a differential role of HPA-axis function, inflammation and metabolic syndrome in melancholic versus atypical depression. Mol Psychiatry 2013;18:692-9.

38. Vancampfort D, Probst M, Knapen J et al. Associations between sedentary behaviour and metabolic parameters in patients with schizophrenia. Psychiatry Res 2012;200:73-8.

39. Dickerson F, Stallings CR, Origoni AE et al. Cigarette smoking among persons with schizophrenia or bipolar disorder in routine clinical settings, 1999-2011. Psychiatr Serv 2013;64:44-50.

40. Bly MJ, Taylor SF, Dalack G et al. Metabolic syndrome in bipolar disorder and schizophrenia: dietary and lifestyle factors compared to the general population. Bipolar Disord 2014;16:277-88.

41. De Hert M, Dekker JM, Wood D et al. Cardiovascular disease and diabetes in people with severe mental illness position statement from the European Psychiatric Association (EPA), supported by the European Association for the Study of Diabetes (EASD) and the European Society of Cardiology (ESC). Eur Psychiatry 2009;24:412-24.

42. McIntyre RS, Alsuwaidan M, Goldstein BI et al. The Canadian Network for Mood and Anxiety Treatments (CANMAT) task force recommendations for the management of patients with mood disorders and comorbid metabolic disorders. Ann Clin Psychiatry 2012;24:69-81.

43. Vancampfort D, De Hert M, Skjerven LH et al. International Organization of Physical Therapy in Mental Health consensus on physical activity within multidisciplinary rehabilitation programmes for minimising cardio-metabolic risk in patients with schizophrenia. Disabil Rehabil 2012;34:1-12.

44. Gierisch JM, Nieuwsma JA, Bradford DW et al. Pharmacologic and behavioral interventions to improve cardiovascular risk factors in adults with serious mental illness: a systematic review and meta-analysis. J Clin Psychiatry 2014;75:424-40.

Psychiatric Emergencies

Basic Rules

1. Medication should not be used simply as an alternative to a physical restraint. This would disregard both, the dignity of another human being and the substantial benefits medication can have if chosen thoughtfully.
2. Form a provisional diagnosis of the most likely cause of the agitation and target the medication to it.
3. Try nonpharmacological approaches, if possible. This primarily includes empathy and thoughtful communication, but can also extend to reducing the noise level, moving to a nicer room with warmer lighting and the team remaining calm themselves.
4. Calm the patient without inducing sleep, if possible.
5. Involve the process of selecting medication and application, such as oral vs intramuscular, to the extent possible. Good communication skills, empathy and respect are key once again.
6. Oral medication should be preferred over intramuscular depot injections, if the patient is compliant.
7. Look for non-psychiatric explanations!

EMPATHIC, RESPECTFUL, THOUGHTFUL COMMUNICATION IS KEY

Non-Psychiatric Causes

Hypoxia and hypoglycemia can lead to delirium that is associated with agitation. In these cases, treating the underlying causes requires the appropriate diagnosis.

Types of Medication

The following types of medication are used most frequently in emergency situations with agitation:

> first-generation antipsychotics
> second-generation antipsychotics, and
> benzodiazepines.

First-Generation Antipsychotics

Typical or first-generation antipsychotics (FGA) have been traditionally used for a long time. They are dopamine antagonists, and, while their effect on dopamine transmission may not be directly responsible for their antipsychotic effect, the FGAs often prove very effective in acute situations.

Phenothiazines

The phenothiazines, a class of medication that includes low-potency antipsychotics such as chlorpromazine (Thorazine®) have a propensity to cause more hypotension, more anticholinergic side effects, and lower the seizure threshold. They are usually not considered first line in the treatment of acute agitated states.

Butyrophenones

Haloperidol is commonly used in psychiatry. Droperidol is not licensed for psychiatric use.

Haloperidol

Haloperidol is the most common used drug to treat acute agitation. It is a highly selective and effective antagonist of the dopamine-2 (D2) receptor.

Haloperidol has minimal effects on vital signs, negligible anticholinergic activity, and minimal interactions with other non-psychiatric medications. However, there are several rare but potentially fatal side effects.

QTc Prolongation
Prolongation of the QT interval can occur, and torsades de points (TdP) have been reported. It seems prudent for physicians to avoid intravenous administration of haloperidol (which is not an FDA-approved route of administration for this medication), especially for patients who are taking other medication that can prolong QTc, who have a preexisting long QTc, or who have other conditions predisposing to TdP or QTc prolongation, such as underlying cardiac abnormalities, electrolyte imbalances (particularly hypokalemia and hypomagnesemia), or hypothyroidism. When haloperidol must be

administered intravenously, it should be administered in conjunction with continuous ECG monitoring and the daily dose be limited.

Extrapyramidal Side Effects (EPS)
In addition to cardiac effects, haloperidol and droperidol carry a risk of inducing acute extrapyramidal side effects (EPS) such as dystonia or neuroleptic malignant syndrome. High doses of these drugs can also cause catatonic reactions due to excessive central dopamine blockade.

One study noted that EPS symptoms occurred in 20% of agitated patients treated with haloperidol alone but in only 6% of agitated patients treated with a combination of haloperidol and lorazepam. [1] This combination treatment was also found to produce more rapid reduction in agitation.

Use in Combination
Studies have found that adding promethazine to haloperidol can similarly reduce the incidence of extrapyramidal side effects. [2] [3] In part because of these studies, haloperidol is frequently administered in combination with another medication such as lorazepam, promethazine, or diphenhydramine. (4) However, using multiple medications to control agitation may increase the risk both of too much sedation and interactions with other medications. In addition, studies on patient preference have indicated that FGAs sometimes cause dysphoria after use. [5] [6] Given that most second-generation antipsychotics have demonstrated good efficacy in treating acute agitation, have low rates of extrapyramidal side effects (see upcoming text), and are subjectively preferred by patients over FGAs, (5,6) the workgroup considers haloperidol to be less preferred than second-generation antipsychotics when an antipsychotic is indicated.

Second-Generation Antipsychotics

Examples of antipsychotics, also called second-generation antipsychotics (SGA) are:

> olanzapine (Zyprexa®)
> ziprasidone (Geodon®)
> aripiprazole (Abilify®)
> risperidone (Risperdal®)
> quetiapine (Seroquel®)

As a class, these medications act as antagonists at the D2 receptor, as do FGAs, but also have comparable or stronger antagonism of other receptor subtypes, particularly 5-HT2A (serotonin) receptors. In addition, this class of medication has actions at other receptor types, such as histamine, norepinephrine, and α-2 receptors. Ziprasidone, for instance, has a high affinity for serotonin receptors compared to D2 receptors, while olanzapine and quetiapine have relatively higher affinities for the histamine receptor.

In general, the SGAs are believed to have a reduced risk of near-term side effects such as dystonia or akathisia. (10-12)

Research appears to show that most members of the class are effective in reducing agitation when compared to placebo and are at least as calming as haloperidol. However, the discussion on the efficacy of SGAs in acute situations continues.

These reviews have generally indicated that most SGAs are equally effective at reducing agitation, with 3 possible exceptions. First, aripiprazole, the only partial D2 agonist approved for agitation, appears slightly less efficacious than other SGAs. Second, research on quetiapine has indicated that while this medication is useful in inpatient settings, it has an unacceptably high risk of orthostatic hypotension in the emergency department where patients are often volume depleted. Third, clozapine is only FDA approved for treatment-resistant schizophrenia and is not generally a first-line agent. Thus, the use of aripiprazole, quetiapine, or clozapine cannot be recommended as first-line agents in the acute control of agitation.

Most published studies of second-generation antipsychotics in agitated patients have not investigated their use either with benzodiazepines or in alcohol-intoxicated patients, and a first-generation antipsychotic may be a safer choice, especially if clinicians anticipate using a benzodiazepine as well.

Benzodiazepines

Benzodiazepines such as diazepam, lorazepam, and clonazepam act on the GABA receptor, the main inhibitory neurotransmitter in the human brain. These medications have a long record of efficacy for agitation and are often preferred by clinicians when the patient is known to be suffering from stimulant intoxication, ethanol withdrawal, or when the etiology of agitation is undetermined. However, in agitation involving psychosis, benzodiazepines alone may only sedate a patient while not addressing the underlying condition that is producing the agitation. In addition, these medications may be overly sedating and have the potential for respiratory depression or hypotension when used parenterally in patients with underlying respiratory conditions or in combination with other CNS depressants such as alcohol. In a minority of patients who chronically abuse stimulants, particularly amphetamines, psychotic symptoms develop as a result of their amphetamine use. In these patients, a first- or second-generation antipsychotic is often useful in addition to, or in place of, a benzodiazepine.

Substance-Induced

Alcohol Intoxication

If possible, reducing environmental stimuli may help to calm the situation even without medication. [7] [8] Often, haloperidol is used as first choice for alcohol intoxication induced agitation. There is also the potential for clinically significant respiratory depression when benzodiazepines are administered to alcohol-intoxicated patients, as both agents are central nervous system (CNS) depressants [9], although it is not entirely clear how significant this is in practice. Nevertheless, the use of haloperidol is generally preferred to the use of benzodiazepines.

Medication to treat agitation associated with alcohol intoxication should be used sparingly if at all. If medication is required, benzodiazepines should be avoided because of the potential to compound the risk of respiratory depression. Thus, antipsychotics are preferred. Haloperidol has the longest track record of safety and efficacy and has minimal effects on respiration. Second-generation antipsychotics, such as olanzapine and risperidone, have not been well studied for alcohol intoxication but may be a reasonable alternative to haloperidol for agitation in the context of alcohol intoxication. Of note, it is important to distinguish agitation secondary to alcohol intoxication versus agitation secondary to alcohol withdrawal, as benzodiazepines are preferred over antipsychotics in alcohol withdrawal. Agitation in a chronic alcohol user who exhibits features of delirium, such as tachycardia, diaphoresis, tremors, and a low or undetectable alcohol blood level, should be presumed to be due to withdrawal and treated accordingly.

Drugs

For intoxication with most recreational drugs, especially stimulants, benzodiazepines are generally considered first-line agents. [13] A minority of chronic amphetamine users develop psychotic symptoms from their amphetamine use. [14] In these patients, a second-generation antipsychotic may be useful in addition to a benzodiazepine.

Psychiatric Illness

Psychosis

Antipsychotics are preferred over benzodiazepines because they address the underlying psychosis. Second-generation antipsychotics can also be mood stabilizing in individuals suffering from a bipolar disorder.

Second-generation antipsychotics with supportive data for their use in acute agitation are preferred over haloperidol either alone or with an adjunctive medication. If the patient is willing to accept oral medication, oral risperidone has the strongest evidence for safety and efficacy, with a smaller number of studies supporting the use of oral antipsychotics such as olanzapine. If the patient cannot cooperate with oral medications, intramuscular ziprasidone or intramuscular olanzapine is preferred for acute control of agitation.

If an initial dose of antipsychotic is insufficient to control agitation, the addition of a benzodiazepine such as lorazepam is preferred to additional doses of the same antipsychotic or to a second antipsychotic.

Delirium

Delirium is a distinct clinical syndrome that frequently is associated with psychosis and agitation. Hallmarks of delirium include

> decreased level of awareness and
> disturbances in attention and cognition (e.g. memory)

that develop over an acute time course (hours to days). The disturbances in cognition and awareness typically fluctuate over hours. Prominence of visual hallucinations or visual perceptual disturbances is a particularly characteristic feature of delirium.

Substance withdrawal

If alcohol or benzodiazepine withdrawal is the suspected cause of delirium, then a benzodiazepine is the agent of choice, [15] since rapid loss of chronic GABA receptor inhibition is implicated in the delirium produced in these circumstances. Clonidine can also be helpful in reducing the sympathetic overdrive of alcohol or benzodiazepine withdrawal, thereby easing delirium and agitation. [16]

If withdrawal from another agent is suspected, replacement of the agent with another that has similar pharmacologic properties should be attempted if safe and appropriate (e.g. nicotine for nicotine withdrawal).

New substance or substance increase

If the recent ingestion of a new agent (or an increased dose of a chronically ingested agent) is the suspected cause of the delirium, then the delirium will be self-limiting. However, agitation may require temporary pharmacologic management.

Medical abnormality

When an underlying medical abnormality (e.g. hypoglycemia, electrolyte imbalance, hypoxia) is the likely cause of delirium, the definitive treatment of the delirium and its associated agitation is correction of the underlying medical condition.

Other reason

If immediate pharmacologic control of agitation is needed in a patient with delirium that is not due to alcohol, benzodiazepine withdrawal, or sleep deprivation, second-generation antipsychotics are the preferred agents. Haloperidol is also acceptable in low doses. [17] Benzodiazepines should be generally avoided because they can exacerbate the delirium. [18]

Agitation from Unknown or Multiple Reasons

If medication is needed to control agitation in a non-delirious patient for whom the underlying etiology of the agitation is not clear, there is little in the way of formal evidence to guide the decision of which agent to use. In patients who do not display psychosis (hallucinations, delusional thinking, paranoia), a benzodiazepine is recommended as first-line treatment. An antipsychotic is recommended in patients who are displaying psychotic features.

Generally, the most important tool is to communicate with the patient and, if possible, establish a working relationship. This helps all involved and prevents misunderstandings

References

1. Battaglia J, Moss S, Rush J, et al. Haloperidol, lorazepam, or both for psychotic agitation: a multicenter, prospective, double-blind, emergency department study. Am J Emerg Med. 1997;15:335–340. [PubMed]

2. Raveendran NS, Tharyan P, Alexander J, et al. TREC-India II Collaborative Group. Rapid tranquillisation in psychiatric emergency settings in India: pragmatic randomised controlled trial of intramuscular olanzapine versus intramuscular haloperidol plus promethazine. BMJ. 2007;335:865–873.

3. Huf G, Alexander J, Allen MH, et al. Haloperidol plus promethazine for psychosis-induced aggression.Cochrane Database Syst Rev. 2009. 3:CD005146.

4. MacDonald K, Wilson MP, Minassian A, et al. A retrospective analysis of intramuscular haloperidol and olanzapine in the treatment of agitation in drug- and alcohol-using patients. Gen Hosp Psychiatry.2010;32:443–445.

5. Lambert M, Schimmelmann BG, Karow A, et al. Subjective well-being and initial dysphoric reaction under antipsychotic drugs—concepts, measurement and clinical relevance. Pharmacopsychiatry. 2003;36((suppl 3)):S181–S190.

6. Karow A, Schnedler D, Naber D. What would the patient choose: subjective comparison of atypical and typical neuroleptics. Pharmacopsychiatry. 2006;39:47–51.

7. Vilke GM, Wilson MP. Agitation: what every emergency physician should know. Emerg Med Rep.2009;30:233–244.

8. Allen MH, Currier GW, Carpenter D, et al. Expert Consensus Panel for Behavioral Emergencies 2005. The Expert Consensus Guideline Series: treatment of behavioral emergencies 2005. J Psychiatr Pract. 2005. pp. 5-108

9. Martel M, Sterzinger A, Miner J, et al. Management of acute undifferentiated agitation in the emergency department: a randomized double-blind trial of droperidol, ziprasidone, and midazolam. Acad Emerg Med.2005;12:1167–1172.

10. Correll CU, Schenk EM. Tardive dyskinesia and new antipsychotics. Curr Opin Psychiatry.2008;21:151–156

11. Dolder CR, Jeste DV. Incidence of tardive dyskinesia with typical versus atypical antipsychotics in very high risk patients. Biol Psychiatry. 2003;53:1142–1145.

12. Kane JM. Tardive dyskinesia rates with atypical antipsychotics in adults: prevalence and incidence. J Clin Psychiatry. 2004;65((suppl 9)):16–20.

13. Ricuarte GA, McCann UD. Recognition and management of complications of new recreational drug use.Lancet. 2005;365:2137–2145.

14. Shoptaw SJ, Kao U, Ling W. Treatment for amphetamine psychosis. Cochrane Database Syst Rev.2009. 1:CD003026.

15. Amato L, Minozzi S, Vecchi S, et al. Benzodiazepines for alcohol withdrawal. Cochrane Database Syst Rev. 2010. 3:CD005063.

16. Muzyk AJ, Fowler JA, Norwood DK, et al. Role of α2-agonists in the treatment of acute alcohol withdrawal. Ann Pharmacother. 2011;45:649–657.

17. Lonergan E, Britton AM, Luxenberg J. Antipsychotics for delirium. Cochrane Database Syst Rev. 2007. 2:CD005594.

18. Clegg A, Young JB. Which medications to avoid in people at risk of delirium: a systematic review. Age Ageing. 2011;40:23–29.

QT Prolongation

Prolongation of the electrocardiographic QT interval is an established risk factor for torsades de pointes (TdP), (1) a malignant ventricular arrhythmia, though the relationship between prolonged QT and TdP is complex. (2) A variety of psychiatric medications have been linked to lengthening of this cardiac interval. (1) Especially in patients who are at a greater risk of heart arrhythmias, it is open to be aware of these possible complications when prescribing psychiatric medication.

Clinicians should be aware of the myriad risk factors for QTc prolongation in their patients and should be mindful of these when prescribing psychotropic medications. Unfortunately, although a link exists between QTc and TdP, this link is neither linear nor straightforward.

500 ms

Most experts do agree that a QTc above 500 ms represents a risk factor for TdP.

Antidepressants

Selective serotonin reuptake inhibitors (SSRIs)

With respect to antidepressants, SSRIs are probably generally safe in patients with risk factors for prolonged QTc. Citalopram, however, in at-risk patients might increase the propensity for QTc prolongation in a dose-dependent manner. The International Registry for Drug-Induced Arrhythmias Arizona Classification now lists citalopram on its "Torsades List," escitalopram on its "Possible Torsades List," and paroxetine, fluoxetine and sertraline on its "Conditional Torsades List." (65)

Clinically, one reasonable approach may be to use sertraline for patients with cardiac disease and/or risk factors for QTc prolongation, given that this agent has few drug–drug interactions, has not been consistently linked to QTc prolongation, and has been the most studied agent in cardiac patients. (30)

Other SSRIs can be used in this population, especially if patients have current or prior good response to a specific agent.

Escitalopram

Over the years, case reports have appeared linking all of the SSRIs except paroxetine to QTc prolongation and, in some instances, to TdP. (3-7) However, case reports by their nature are anecdotal and nonsystematic, and many of these specific reports have suffered from incomplete data, such as concomitant medical illness or method of QT measurement.

Two prospective studies found that citalopram 60 mg daily for 4 weeks had no effect on the QTc interval of healthy male volunteers, and an additional study determined that citalopram 40 mg daily for 12 weeks resulted in no QTc prolongation in depressed patients with coronary artery disease. (8-10) However, cumulative evidence in later years suggested that some SSRIs, particularly citalopram, may have a predictable negative effect on the QTc interval. A randomized, multi-center, double-blind, placebo-controlled, crossover study for 40 mg citalopram estimated the prolongation of the QTc interval at 12.6 ms, based on serum concentrations. (11) The Food and Drug Administration (FDA) recommended in August 2011 to limit the maximum daily dose of citalopram to 40 mg (20 mg in patients with hepatic impairment or those older than 60 years) because of the increased risk of QTc prolongation at higher doses. (11) Citalopram is also "not recommended" for patients with congenital LQTS and there is a recommendation to discontinue citalopram in any patient with a QTc interval greater than 500ms. (12) A later study suggested that citalopram was associated with out-of-hospital cardiac arrest, though it did not examine the QTc interval specifically. (13)

Escitalopram is one of the two racemates of citalopram, and one might expect it to carry similar risks as the citalopram in regard to prolonging the QT interval. However, a thorough QT study of escitalopram (n=113), essentially identical to that performed for citalopram, found dose-dependent but substantially less marked increases of QTc associated with escitalopram (4.5 and 10.7 ms for 10 and 30 mg, respectively). (14) In general, QTc prolongation rates may be relatively low with citalopram, even in overdose, as a study of 215 patients with a citalopram overdose found that 32% had a QTc over 440 ms and 2% had a QTc over 500 ms. (15)

Other Selective Serotonin Reuptake Inhibitors

At least 13 studies designed to measure an effect on the QTc interval, including at least five studies involving fluoxetine and five involving paroxetine, failed to show any association between these agents and QTc prolongation. (16-28) All this suggests that citalopram may be separate from other SSRIs in its propensity to prolong the QTc interval.

Serotonin and norepinephrine reuptake inhibitors (SNRIs)

There has been at least one case in which venlafaxine was linked to QT prolongation, but to the author's knowledge there are no systematic studies which have shown a significant QT prolongation for either venlafaxine or duloxetine.

Tricyclic Antidepressants

All tricyclic antidepressants (TCAs) can cause prolongation of the QTc interval through sodium channel blockade, which leads to QRS widening, and through calcium channel blockade. (32)

TCAs generally only pose a significant risk of ventricular arrhythmia to patients with preexisting cardiac disease, including intraventricular conduction disease or ischemic heart disease. (33) Like other QTc-prolonging medications, they also block the IKr channel.

A systematic review in 2004 found amitriptyline and maprotiline to be most commonly implicated in TdP. (34) Clomipramine may be associated with the least QTc prolongation. (35)

Noradrenergic and specific serotonergic antidepressants (NaSSAs)

Mirtazapine

In a study on 103 patients who had ingested mirtazapine in overdose, 16% had prolongation of the QTc over 440 ms, with none over 500 ms. (36)

Norepinephrine-dopamine reuptake inhibitor (NDRI)

Bupropion

Some have reported prolongation of the QT interval in the setting of bupropion overdose, though this finding may be confounded by tachycardia. (37) No studies seem to have linked therapeutic doses of bupropion to QTc prolongation.

Serotonin antagonist and reuptake inhibitors (SARIs)

Trazodone

Trazodone has been associated with mild QTc prolongation, mainly in the setting of overdose. [35]

Antipsychotics

Antipsychotic medications have long been known to have the potential to cause QTc interval prolongation and TdP. Retrospective and cohort studies have linked antipsychotic use with sudden cardiac death, and most antipsychotic medications have been shown to cause some degree of QT prolongation. (68-70) As with citalopram, the mechanism by which this occurs is thought to involve blockade of IKr channels.

First-Generation Antipsychotics

In general, low potency typical antipsychotics are thought to carry a greater risk than high-potency agents, and this risk is thought to be dose related. (5)

Thioridazine

Thioridazine was the first antipsychotic medication associated with QTc prolongation and TdP, (36) and is still commonly associated with it. In a randomized, prospective study evaluating the effects of QTc on medically healthy individuals with psychotic disorders, it showed the greatest prolongation of the QTc compared with ziprasidone, risperidone, olanzapine, quetiapine (750 mg/d), or haloperidol (15 mg/d). (37)

Fluphenazine

Fluphenazine, a high-potency antipsychotic, has been associated with QTc prolongation in patients with schizophrenia. (38)

Haloperidol

Haloperidol has been linked in case reports to QTc prolongation and TdP, though the frequency and magnitude of QTc prolongation is thought to be substantially less than with thioridazine and similar to that with many atypical antipsychotics. (37,39)

In one of the few randomized studies of its effects of QTc, haloperidol (15 mg by mouth daily) led to an average increase in QTc of 7.1 ms, which was less than the prolongation caused by thioridazine or ziprasidone but greater than that caused by olanzapine, risperidone, or quetiapine. (37) In a nearly identical study of the same medications, oral haloperidol 15 mg daily led to an average QTc increase of 4.7 ms, which was less than ziprasidone, olanzapine, risperidone, quetiapine or thioridazine. (39)

Second-Generation Antipsychotics

Atypical antipsychotics also appear to have a risk of QTc interval prolongation, though these agents have only been implicated in the development of TdP in rare case reports and FDA adverse event reports. (40,41)

In elderly patients with dementia, atypical antipsychotics have been associated with mortality related to cardiac events, which has led to an FDA black box warning for these medications. There are less data available about the newest atypical antipsychotics, including aripiprazole, asenapine, paliperidone, and iloperidone. Iloperidone and paliperidone seem to have the highest risk for QTc prolongation, particularly in the presence of 2D6 and 3A4 inhibitors. (51-59) However, there do not appear to be any reported cases of TdP with any of these new medications. (60)

Ziprasidone

Ziprasidone apparently causes the greatest mean QTc prolongation compared with olanzapine, risperidone, and quetiapine. (37,39) Its modest but definite effect on repolarization does not appear to be dose-dependent. (37,39,42) In clinical trials of patients taking therapeutic doses of ziprasidone (i.e., not in overdose), the incidence of QTc prolongation exceeding 500 ms has been estimated at less than 0.06%. (43) Ziprasidone has been associated with TdP in at least two case reports. (44,45)

Olanzapine, Risperidone, Quetiapine

In two randomized, open-label studies, olanzapine, risperidone, and quetiapine were found to have less QTc prolongation than thioridazine and comparable effects to oral haloperidol. (37,39) While these medications all are associated with QTc prolongation, their associations with TdP are less clear. In one large case-control study, atypical antipsychotics were associated with an increased risk of sudden death after controlling for cardiac risk factors, hypokalemia, renal disease, and SSRI use. (46) However, the risk appeared greatest for those patients who were prescribed the medications for the first time within the past 30 days, suggesting that these medications may in some cases have been used for delirium or management of agitation in the setting of medical illness. In a separate, retrospective, population-based cohort study, both typical and atypical antipsychotics were associated with an approximately 2-fold increased risk of sudden cardiac death; similar risk increases were found among all agents examined individually (thioridazine, haloperidol, olanzapine, quetiapine, risperidone, and clozapine). (47)

Clozapine

While clozapine was associated with an increased risk of sudden cardiac death in one study (47), it has only been associated with QTc prolongation in rare case reports, suggesting that another mechanism may be mediating its relationship with sudden cardiac death. (48-50)

Aripiprazole

Aripiprazole has not been associated with significant QTc prolongation, even in the setting of significant medical comorbidity. (31,61)

Mood Stabilizers

Lithium

Lithium in concentrations above 1.2 mmol/L can prolong the QTc interval, though no cases of TdP have been reported. (47)

Anticonvulsants

Anticonvulsant mood stabilizing agents, including

> valproate
> lamotrigine
> carbamazepine, or
> oxcarbazepine,

have not been found to cause QTc prolongation.

Stimulants

There is no strong evidence to suggest that methylphenidate or amphetamines cause clinically significant increases in QTc, (48) while the effects of atomoxetine on QTc remain uncertain.

Benzodiazepines

There is no evidence to suggest that benzodiazepines cause QTc prolongation.

Routine Monitoring

Antidepressants

At this stage, there is no clear rationale for routinely obtaining electrolytes, other labs, or an ECG prior to initiation of an antidepressant. However, this may not apply to patients with substantial risk factors, e.g. significant structural heart disease, including a prior myocardial infarction or a history of non-TdP ventricular arrhythmia. In such a situation, obtaining an ECG, potassium, and magnesium before starting a patient with substantial risk factors for TdP on citalopram, and before starting any patient with prior TdP on any antidepressant, is recommended. Consulting a cardiologist if in doubt is advisable.

Antipsychotics

Low-potency typical antipsychotics, IV haloperidol, and ziprasidone may carry the highest risk, though there is limited evidence for actual adverse QTc related outcomes with ziprasidone.

Though limited evidence suggests that some atypical antipsychotics (i.e., olanzapine) may be less likely to prolong the QTc interval, this has not been rigorously studied. For patients with risk factors for QTc prolongation, QTc should be assessed at baseline and intermittently post-initiation when prescribing any antipsychotic.

For patients receiving parenteral haloperidol in the hospital for agitation or psychosis, it is prudent to monitor QTc at baseline, and then at least daily, and sometimes more frequently depending on the risk. If the QTc extends beyond 500 ms, potassium/magnesium should be repleted and the patient's medication regimen should be examined for other potential QTc-prolonging agents, with consideration given to holding haloperidol until the QTc has dropped below 500 ms. Other options to manage acute agitation should be considered, including valproate, trazodone, and alternative antipsychotic agents, with the caveat that none of the antipsychotics typically used to treat agitation in the hospital have zero risk of QTc prolongation. When an alternative antipsychotic medication is used, it often is helpful to choose one which is more sedating (e.g., quetiapine or olanzapine) so that a lower overall dose can be used; this may reduce the risk of QTc prolongation. In some situations, however, the risk of self-injury or harm to others because of severe agitation may outweigh the risk of arrhythmia, suggesting an indication for continuation of IV haloperidol with ongoing close monitoring.

Risk-Benefit Analysis

In all cases, the decision on starting (and continuing) a psychotropic medication in a patient with increased risk for prolonged QTc should involve a careful risk–benefit analysis, taking into account indications for the medication, necessity for immediate treatment, and potential alternative strategies.

References

1. Malik M, Camm AJ: Evaluation of drug-induced QT interval prolongation: implications for drug approval and labeling. Drug Saf 2001; 24:323–351

2. Alvarez PA, Pahissa J: QT alterations in psychopharmoacology: proven candidates and suspects. Curr Drug Saf 2010; 5:97–104

3. Catalano G, Catalano MC, Epstein MA, Tsambiras PE: QTc interval prolongation associated with citalopram overdose: a case report and literature review. Clin Neuropharmacol 2001; 24:158–162

4. Nykamp DL, Blackmon CL, Schmidt PE, Roberson AG: QTc prolongation associated with combination therapy of

levofloxacin, imipramine and fluoxetine. Ann Pharmacother 2005; 39:543–546

5. Brendel DH, Bodkin JA, Yang JM: Massive sertraline overdose. Ann Emerg Med 2000; 36:524–526

6. Brzozowska A, Werner B: Observation of QTc prolongation in an adolescent girl during fluvoxamine pharmacotherapy. J Child Adolesc Psychopharmacol 2009; 19:591–592

7. Yuksel FV, Tuzer V, Goka E: Escitalopram intoxication. Eur Psychiatry 2005; 20:82

8. Slavícek J, Paclt I, Hamplová J, Kittnar O, Trefný Z, Horácek BM: Antidepressant drugs and heart electrical field. Physiol Res 1998; 47:297–300

9. Rasmussen SL, Overø KF, Tanghøj P: Cardiac safety of citalopram: prospective trials and retrospective analyses. J Clin Psychopharmacol 1999; 19:407–415

10. Lespérance F, Frasure-Smith N, Koszycki D, Laliberté MA, van Zyl LT, Baker B, et al: Effects of citalopram and interpersonal psychotherapy on depression in patients with coronary artery disease: the Canadian cardiac randomized evaluation of antidepressant and psychotherapy efficacy (CREATE) trial. JAMA 2007; 297:367–379

11. US Food and Drug Administration: FDA safety communication: abnormal heart rhythms associated with high doses of Celexa (citalopram hydrobromide). http://www.fda.gov/Drugs/DrugSafety/ucm269086.htm

12. US Food and Drug Administration: FDA safety communication: revised recommendations for (citalopram hydrobromide) related to a potential risk of abnormal heart rhythms with high doses. http://www.fda.gov/Drugs/DrugSafety/ucm297391.htm

13. Weeke P, Jensen A, Folke F, Gislason GS, Olesen JB, Andersson C, et al: Antidepressant use and risk of out-of-hospital cardiac arrest: a nationwide case-time-control study. Clin Pharmacol Ther 2012; 92:72–79

14. Evaluation of the effects of sequential multiple-dose regimens of escitalopram on cardiac repolarization in healthy subjects. http://www.forestclinicaltrials.com/CTR/CTRController/CTRViewPDf?_file_idscsr/SCSR_SCT-PK- 21_final.pdf.

15. Waring WS, Graham A, Gray J, Wilson AD, Howell C, Bateman DN: Evaluation of a QT nomogram for risk assessment after antidepressant overdose. Br J Clin Pharmacol 2010; 70: 881–885

16. Zemrak WR, Kenna GA: Association of antipsychotic and antidepressant drugs with Q-T interval prolongation. Am J Health Syst Pharm 2008; 65:1029–1038

17. Abramson DW, Quinn DK, Stern TA: Methadone-associated QTc prolongation: a case report and review of the literature. Prim Care Companion J Clin Psychiatry 2008; 10:470–476

18. Baker B, Dorian P, Sandor P, Shapiro C, Schell C, Mitchell J, et al: Electrocardiographic effects of fluoxetine and doxepin in patients with major depressive disorder. J Clin Psychopharmacol 1997; 17:15–21

19. Strik JJ, Honig A, Lousberg R, Cheriex EC, Tuynman-Qua HG, Kujpers PM, et al: Efficacy and safety of fluoxetine in the treatment of patients with major depression after first myocardial infarction: findings from a double-blind, placebo-controlled trial Psychsom Med 2000; 62(6):783–789

20. Roose SP, Glassman AH, Attia E, Woodring S, Giardina EG, Bigger JT Jr: Cardiovascular effects of fluoxetine in depressed patients with heart disease. Am J Psychiatry 1998; 155:660–665

21. Pohl R, Balon R, Jayaraman A, Doll RG, Yeragani V: Effect of fluoxetine, pemoline and placebo on heart period and QT variability in normal humans. J Psychosom Res 2003; 55:247–251

22. Edwards JG, Goldie A, Papayanni-Papasthatis S: Effect of paroxetine on the electrocardiogram. Psychopharmacology 1989; 97:96–98

23. Kuhs H, Rudolf GAE: Cardiovascular effects of paroxetine. Psychopharmacology 1990; 102:379–382

24. Nelson JC, Pritchett YL, Martynov O, Yu JY, Mallinckrodt CH, Detke MJ: The safety and tolerability of duloxetine compared with paroxetine and placebo: a pooled analysis of 4 clinical trials. Prim Care Companion J Clin Psychiatry 2006; 8:212–219

25. Roose SP, Laghrissi-Thode F, Kennedy JS, Nelson JC, Bigger JT Jr, Pollock BG, et al: Comparison of paroxetine and nortriptyline in depressed patients with ischemic heart disease. JAMA 1998; 279:287–291

26. Fisch C, Knoebel SB: Electrocardiographic findings in sertraline depression trials. Drug Investigation 1992; 4(4):305–312

27. Glassman AH, O'Connor CM, Califf RM, Swedberg K, Schwartz P, Bigger JT Jr, et al: Sertraline treatment of major depression in patients with acute MI or unstable angina. JAMA 2002; 288:701–709

28. Yeragani VK, Pohl R, Kampala VC, Balon R, Ramesh C, Srinivasan K: Effects of nortriptyline and paroxetine on QT variability in patients with panic disorder depress. Anxiety 2000; 11:126-130

29. Letsas K, Korantzopoulos P, Pappas L, Evangelou D, Efremidis M, Kardaras F: QT interval prolongation

associated with venlafaxine administration. Int J Cardiol 2006; 109:116–117

30. Jiang W, O'Connor C, Silva SG, Kuchibhatla M, Cuffe MS, Callwood DD, et al: Safety and efficacy of sertraline for depression in patients with CHF (SADHART-CHF): a randomized, double-blind, placebo-controlled trial of sertraline for major depression with congestive heart failure. Am Heart J 2008; 156:437–444

31. Belgamwar RB, El-Sayeh HG: Aripiprazole versus placebo for schizophrenia. Cochrane Database Syst Rev 2011; 8:CD00 6622:CD006622

32. Vieweg WV, Wood MA: Tricyclic antidepressants, QT interval prolongation, and torsades de pointes. Psychosomatics 2004; 45:371–377

33. Glassman AH: Cardiovascular effects of tricyclic antidepressants. Annu Rev Med 1984; 35:503–511

34. Vieweg WV, Wood MA: Tricyclic antidepressants, QT interval prolongation, and torsades de pointes. Psychosomatics 2004; 45:371–377

35. Wenzel-Seifert K, Wittmann M, Haen E: QTc prolongation by psychotropic drugs and the risk of torsades de pointes. Dtsch Arztebl Int 2011; 108(41):687–693

36. Kelly HG, Fay JE, Laverty SG: Thioridazine hydrochloride (Mellaril): its effect on the electrocardiogram and a report

of two fatalities with electrocardiographic abnormalities. Can Med Assoc J 1963; 89:546–554

37. Isbister GK, Balit CR: Bupropion overdose: QTc prolongation and its clinical significance. Ann Pharmacother 2003; 37:999–1002

38. Chong SA, Mythily, Lum A, Goh HY, Chan YH: Prolonged QTc intervals in medicated patients with schizophrenia. Hum Psychopharmacol 2003; 18:647–649

39. FDA. Briefing Document for Zeldox Capsules (Ziprasidone). New York: Pfizer Inc, July 18 2000; 116

40. Vieweg WV, Schneider RK, Wood MA: Torsade de pointes in a patient with complex medical and psychiatric conditions receiving low-dose quetiapine. Acta Psychiatr Scand 2005; 112: 318–322; author reply:322

41. Poluzzi E, Raschi E, Moretti U, De Ponti F: Drug-induced torsades de pointes: data mining of the public version of the FDA Adverse Event Reporting System (AERS). Pharmacoepidemiol Drug Saf 2009; 18(6):512–518

42. Miceli JJ, Tensfeldt TG, Shiovitz T, Anziano R, O'Gorman C, Harrigan RH: Effects of oral ziprasidone and oral haloperidol on QTc interval in patients with schizophrenia or schizoaffective disorder. Pharmacotherapy 2010; 30:127–135

43. Klein-Schwartz W, Lofton AL, Benson BE, Spiller HA, Crouch BI: Prospective observational multi-poison center study of ziprasidone exposures. Clin Toxicol 2007; 45:782–786

44. Heinrich TW, Biblo LA, Schneider J: Torsades de pointes associated with ziprasidone. Psychosomatics 2006; 47:264–268

45. Manini AF, Hoffman RS, Nelson LS: Delayed torsade de pointes (TdP) associated with ziprasidone overdose [abstract]. Clin Toxicol (Phila) 2007; 45:366

46. Poluzzi E, Raschi E, Moretti U, De Ponti F: Drug-induced torsades de pointes: data mining of the public version of the FDA Adverse Event Reporting System (AERS). Pharmacoepidemiol Drug Saf 2009; 18(6):512–518

47. Hsu CH, Liu PY, Chen JH, Yeh TL, Tsai HY, Lin LJ: Electrocardiographic abnormalities as predictors for over-range lithium levels. Cardiology 2007; 103:101–106

48. Stiefel G, Besag FMC: Cardiovascular effects of methylphenidate, amphetamines and atomoxetine in the treatment of attention-deficit hyperactivity disorder. Drug Saf 2010; 33:821–842

49. Stöllberger C, Huber JO, Finsterer J: Antipsychotic drugs and QT prolongation. Int Clin Psychopharmacol 2005; 20:243–251

50. Warner B, Hoffmann P: Investigation of the potential of clozapine to cause torsade de pointes. Adverse Drug React Toxicol Rev 2002; 21:189–203

51. Citrome L: Iloperidone: a clinical overview. J Clin Psychiatry 2011; 72(Suppl 1):19–23

52. Fanapt (Iloperidone) [package insert]. East Hanover, NJ: Novartis Pharmaceuticals Corp., 2012

53. Weiden PJ, Cutler AJ, Polymeropoulos MH, Wolfgang CD: Safety profile of iloperidone: a pooled analysis of 6-week acute-phase pivotal trials. J Clin Psychopharmacol 2008; 28(Suppl 1):S12–S19

54. Invega, (paliperidone) [package insert]. Titusville, NJ: JanssenPharmaceuticals, Inc.; 2011

55. Hough DW, Natarajan J, Vandebosch A, Rossenu S, Kramer M, Eerdekens M: Evaluation of the effect of paliperidone extended release and quetiapine on corrected QT intervals: a randomized, double-blind, placebo-controlled study. Int Clin Psychopharmacol 2011; 26:25–34

56. Citrome L: Asenapine for schizophrenia and bipolar disorder: a review of the efficacy and safety profile for this newly approved sublingually absorbed second-generation antipsychotic. Int J Clin Pract 2009; 63:1762–1784

57. Saphris: (Asenapine) [package insert]. Whitehouse Station, NJ: Merck, Sharpe and Dohme Corp. 2012

58. Latudalurasidone) [package insert]. Marlborough, MA: Sunovion Pharmaceuticals, Inc. 2012

59. Potkin SG, Ogasa M, Cucchiaro J, Loebel A: Double-blind comparison of the safety and efficacy of lurasidone and ziprasidone in clinically stable outpatients with schizophrenia or schizoaffective disorder. Schizophr Res 2011; 132: 101–107

60. Vieweg WV, Wood MA: Tricyclic antidepressants, QT interval prolongation, and torsades de pointes. Psychosomatics 2004; 45:371–377

61. Muzyk AJ, Rivelli SK, Gagliardi JP, Revollo JY, Jiang W: A retrospective study exploring the effects of intramuscular aripiprazole on QTc change in agitated medically ill patients J. Clin Psychopharmacol 2011; 31:532–534

Serotonin Syndrome

Serotonin syndrome is a drug induced syndrome characterized by a cluster of dose related adverse effects that are due to increased serotonin concentrations in the central nervous system. It can range from mild to severe, but it is assumed to depend on rising serotonin levels [1] [2], and thus on more serotonergic activity. In a broader sense, the term 'serotonin toxicity' is used to describe related undesired effects that are caused by serotonergic agents.

In the central nervous system, serotonin is a neurotransmitter with many effects, including modification of mood, sleep, vomiting, and pain. Many drugs influence serotonergic neurotransmission, including some antidepressants, appetite suppressants, analgesics, sedatives, antipsychotics, anxiolytics, antimigraine drugs, and antiemetics. [1] [2]

Serotonergic Effects

Only drugs that can increase serotonin levels seem to cause the serotonin syndrome. This includes, for example the selective serotonin reuptake inhibitors (SSRIs), serotonin and norepinephrine reuptake inhibitors (SNRIs), tricyclic antidepressants (TCAs), second generation antipsychotics (SGAs), and a number of other psychiatric and non-psychiatric drugs.

5-HT2 receptor agonists

Severe or life-threatening effects (rigidity and hyperthermia) seem to result only from stimulation of 5-HT2 receptors.

5-HT1A, 5-HT1D, 5-HT3 receptor agonists
serotonin antagonists

Antipsychotics, anxiolytics, antimigraine drugs, and antiemetics, which are serotonin antagonists or have effects on other specific receptors (5-HT1A, 5-HT1D, 5-HT3), do not carry a significant risk of serotonin toxicity. [1] [4] [6]

Drug Changes

Serotonergic adverse effects in therapeutic use will not progress to severe toxicity in the absence of dose escalation or drug interactions. For some patients with a good therapeutic response, continuation of the drug at the same or a lower dose may be justifiable.

There are usually only three situations involving medication which may trigger a serotonin syndrome:

- starting serotonergic medication
- increasing serotonergic medication
- adding medication

However, some drugs may have long lasting activity, such as an irreversible MAO inhibitor, or a long-half life, such as fluoxetine, which can still trigger a serotonin syndrome after they have been discontinued.

Combinations

Severe toxicity usually occurs only with a combination of two or more serotonergic drugs (even when each is at a therapeutic dose), one of which is generally a monoamine oxidase inhibitor. [1] [3]

Overdose

Moderate toxicity has been reported with an overdose of a single drug and occasionally from increasing therapeutic doses. [1] [3] [4] Moderate serotonin toxicity appears to occur in about 15% of SSRI overdoses. [5]

Serotonin Toxicity

Drug classes that are implicated in serotonin toxicity are largely restricted to [4]

- Serotonin precursors
- serotonin agonists
- drugs causing serotonin release
- serotonin reuptake inhibitors
- monoamine oxidase inhibitors

Certain herbal medicines can also be included. St John's Wort, for example, has serotonergic effects.

Although case series showed moderate serotonin toxicity occurred in 15% of SSRI overdoses, there were no severe cases. [5] Serotonin toxicity did not occur in overdoses of the reversible monoamine oxidase inhibitor moclobemide alone. However, if a second serotonergic drug was ingested, serotonin toxicity was nearly always present and was severe in about half of these cases. [15]

In some other cases, the symptoms remind clearly of a serotonin syndrome, but the mechanism remains unclear. [7] These drugs generally have effects on other neurotransmitters and may have secondary effects on serotonin release or reuptake.

Severe Toxicity

Severe serotonin toxicity is characterized by a rapidly rising temperature and rigidity. The diagnosis can be made on clinical grounds.

Mild Toxicity

Patients taking therapeutic SSRIs commonly have features such as lower limb hyperreflexia or a few beats of ankle clonus without toxicity. One may make a presumptive diagnosis only after exclusion of other explanations, and only if the drug is known to increase serotonin. The diagnosis is further supported if the symptoms stop, once the medication is discontinued.

Symptoms

The classic triad of clinical features are

- neuromuscular excitation (such as clonus, hyperreflexia, myoclonus, rigidity)
- autonomic nervous system excitation (such as hyperthermia, tachycardia), and
- altered mental state (such as agitation, confusion).

These symptoms usually occur within a few hours of ingesting the serotonergic medication.

Hunter Serotonin Toxicity Criteria (HSTC)

Several clinical diagnostic criteria have been used to diagnose serotonin toxicity. The Sternbach criteria were the first suggested, but they were developed from the literature, did not include some of the most important diagnostic features (e.g., clonus), and included a number of non-specific features. They are no longer used.

The HSTC were developed from a large series of overdoses of serotonergic drugs and have now been used in several other studies of therapeutic drug use. These criteria rely on a good focused neurological examination, including assessing tone, clonus, and reflexes.

In the presence of a serotonergic agent, serotonin toxicity exists if ONE of the following criteria is satisfied:

- spontaneous clonus
- inducible clonus AND agitation or diaphoresis
- ocular clonus AND agitation or diaphoresis
- tremor AND hyperreflexia
- hypertonia AND pyrexia (temperature >38°C [>100.4°F]) AND ocular clonus or inducible clonus

One should also be aware of substances such as stimulants and herbal medicines, like St John's wort, ginseng, tryptophan, and pharmaceutical appetite suppressants. Potentially serotonergic are also tramadol, fentanyl, linezolid, and methylene blue.

Differential Diagnosis

There are a number of possible differential diagnoses when presented with these symptoms, such as alcohol or drug withdrawal, non-convulsive seizures, and encephalitis.

Neuroleptic Malignant Syndrome

The key differentiating features are that neuroleptic malignant syndrome is of relatively slow onset over days, and marked by extrapyramidal features and rigidity, but clonus is not a feature.

Prevention

Several systematic reviews clarify the extent to which severe serotonin syndrome may result from drug interactions. [3] [4] [6] [9-11] It is apparent from systematic reviews of case reports [3] [4] [6] [9-11] that nearly all severe serotonin syndromes involve a monoamine oxidase inhibitor. Washout periods should be observed when switching antidepressants. If possible avoid the use of serotonergic drugs for non-psychiatric conditions (such as tramadol for analgesia).

Interactions of an SSRI with any monoamine oxidase inhibitor might be lethal and should be avoided at all cost. However, interactions with other serotonin reuptake inhibitors are likely to be minor (additive effect), and interactions with serotonin releasing agents (such as amphetamines) might even attenuate toxicity.18

Many listed interactions—such as with carbamazepine, most tricyclic and atypical antidepressants, [4] [12] and triptans [6] —have little or no evidence to support the contention that serotonergic effects are increased by co-administration. However, clomipramine and imipramine are much more serotonergic than other tricyclic antidepressants and have caused serotonin toxicity.

Patients also need to be aware of the potential for serious drug interactions, especially given the existence of over the counter drugs and herbal medicines with serotonergic activity.

Some individuals seem to be more susceptible, but it is unclear if pharmacokinetic (such as decreased drug metabolism) or pharmacodynamic (such as serotonin receptor polymorphism) differences explain this, and strong consistent pharmacogenetic associations have not been found. [19] No evidence has been found to support theories that potent dietary monoamine oxidase inhibitor compounds are a cause of serotonin toxicity in highly susceptible individuals. [20]

Treatment

Mild to moderate cases

Serotonin syndrome in mild to moderate cases usually resolves in one to three days after stopping the serotonergic drugs.

Severe cases

Intensive support care is needed. Severe toxicity is a medical emergency and may be complicated by severe hyperthermia, rhabdomyolysis, disseminated intravascular coagulation, and adult respiratory distress syndrome. [17]

Supportive care largely consists of sedation as required. Ensuring adequate hydration and careful monitoring of temperature, pulse, blood pressure, and urine output are necessary. Preventing hyperthermia and subsequent multiorgan failure is a key goal in severe serotonin toxicity.

Body temperature

In animal models lowering temperature also indirectly down regulated 5HT2A receptors in the central nervous system and reduced serotonin levels.2 Sedation to reduce muscle hyperactivity (such as midazolam infusion or oral diazepam), active cooling (fans with water sprays, ice packs, or cooling blankets), and even paralysis and ventilation may be useful in severe cases. Serotonin antagonists and in particular 5HT2A receptor antagonists reduce hyperthermia and other severe manifestations in animal studies. [1] [2] [8]

Medication

For severe serotonin toxicity, intravenous chlorpromazine is the most commonly used serotonin antagonist, but intravenous fluid loading is essential to prevent hypotension. [8] Oral cyproheptadine has been used to treat moderate serotonin toxicity, with doses of 8-16 mg up to a daily maximum of 32 mg. Whether its sedative or serotonin antagonist effects are more important remains unclear.

In moderate serotonin toxicity agitation is generally the most troublesome symptom, and sedation with oral diazepam may be all that is required.

Prognosis

There are no clinical trials or other strong evidence supporting the mentioned treatment approaches, [8] but recovery is apparently usual and mortality low (<1%) when they are applied. [5] [15]

References

1. Isbister GK, Buckley NA. The pathophysiology of serotonin toxicity in animals and humans: implications for diagnosis and treatment. Clin Neuropharmacol 2005;28:205-14.

2. Krishnamoorthy S, Ma Z, Zhang G, Wei J, Auerbach SB, Tao R. Involvement of 5-HT2A receptors in the serotonin (5-HT) syndrome caused by excessive 5-HT efflux in rat brain. Basic Clin Pharmacol Toxicol 2010;107:830-41.

3. Gillman PK. CNS toxicity involving methylene blue: the exemplar for understanding and predicting drug interactions that precipitate serotonin toxicity. J Psychopharmacol 2011;25:429-36.

4. Gillman PK. A review of serotonin toxicity data: implications for the mechanisms of antidepressant drug action. Biol Psychiatry 2006;59:1046-51.

5. Isbister GK, Bowe SJ, Dawson A, Whyte IM. Relative toxicity of selective serotonin reuptake inhibitors (SSRIs) in overdose. J Toxicol Clin Toxicol 2004;42:277-85.

6. Evans RW, Tepper SJ, Shapiro RE, Sun-Edelstein C, Tietjen GE. The FDA alert on serotonin syndrome with use of triptans combined with selective serotonin reuptake inhibitors or selective serotonin-norepinephrine reuptake inhibitors: American Headache Society position paper. Headache 2010;50:1089-99.

7. Karunatilake H, Buckley NA. Serotonin syndrome induced by fluvoxamine and oxycodone. Ann Pharmacother 2006;40:155-7.

8. Isbister GK, Buckley NA, Whyte IM. Serotonin toxicity: a practical approach to diagnosis and treatment. Med J Aust 2007;187:361-5.

9. Gillman PK. Is there sufficient evidence to suggest cyclobenzaprine might be implicated in causing serotonin toxicity? Am J Emerg Med 2009;27:509-10.

10. Gillman PK. Monoamine oxidase inhibitors, opioid analgesics and serotonin toxicity. Br J Anaesth 2005;95:434-41.

11. Ramsey TD, Lau TT, Ensom MH. Serotonergic and adrenergic drug interactions associated with linezolid: a critical review and practical management approach. Ann Pharmacother 2013;47:543-60.

12. Gillman PK. Tricyclic antidepressant pharmacology and therapeutic drug interactions updated. Br J Pharmacol 2007;151:737-48.

13. Dunkley EJ, Isbister GK, Sibbritt D, Dawson AH, Whyte IM. The Hunter serotonin toxicity criteria: simple and accurate diagnostic decision rules for serotonin toxicity. QJM 2003;96:635-42.

14. Sternbach H. The serotonin syndrome. Am J Psychiatry 1991;148:705.

15. Isbister GK, Hackett LP, Dawson AH, Whyte IM, Smith AJ. Moclobemide poisoning: toxicokinetics and occurrence of serotonin toxicity. Br J Clin Pharmacol 2003;56:441-50.

16. Buckley NA, Dawson AH, Whyte IM. Hypertox. Assessment and treatment of poisoning. 2013. www.hypertox.com.

17. Neuvonen PJ, Pohjola-Sintonen S, Tacke U, Vuori E. Five fatal cases of serotonin syndrome after moclobemide-citalopram or moclobemide-clomipramine overdoses. Lancet 1993;342:1419.

18. Liechti ME, Vollenweider FX. The serotonin uptake inhibitor citalopram reduces acute cardiovascular and vegetative effects of 3,4-methylenedioxymethamphetamine ('ecstasy') in healthy volunteers. J Psychopharmacol 2000;14:269-74.

19. Porcelli S, Drago A, Fabbri C, Gibiino S, Calati R, Serretti A. Pharmacogenetics of antidepressant response. J Psychiatry Neurosci 2011;36:87-113.

20. Dixon Clarke SE, Ramsay RR. Dietary inhibitors of monoamine oxidase A. J Neural Transm 2011;118:1031-41.

The Combination with Psychotherapy

As mentioned, psychiatric drugs can support psychotherapy. Psychotherapy, if done correctly, is always more specific than any chemical compound that floods the brain and affects all information transmission mediated by a certain class of neurotransmitters and receptors. But in order for psychotherapy to work, the individual has to be receptive to the information and the interaction offered by the therapist, and if the condition is severe or in situations of psychological stress this may not be possible without proper medication.

If a patient suffering from depression has lost any motivation to communicate, psychotherapy may only be of limited effectiveness. However, even in these cases, one should not disconnect from the patient or let the patient feel disconnected, which tends to make the depression worse.

Medication as a Bridge to Help Communicating

Medication should be viewed as a tool that ultimately helps regain the capability to partake in interactions. This allows the communication process to take place and bring about beneficial changes.

If a patient is completely detached from reality because of a psychosis or from the after-effects of a severe trauma, medication may help to establish a rapport between patient and therapist.

Assessment of Medication

Over the medium- and long-run the indication for medication, just like for psychotherapy, needs to be evaluated regularly. Even therapists who do not prescribe medication should develop an eye for the dynamics of medication and be in contact with the prescriber, so that needed changes can be made early on.

Communication-Focused Therapy (CFT)

CFT was developed by the author to focus on the communication process as the key element in the 'talking cure'. Information in the form of meaningful messages flows back and forth between the therapist and the patient. Novel information, whether from inside or from the therapist, which the patient sees as relevant automatically changes the perspective and understanding of the patient about himself and the world, while the practice in the communication with the therapist facilitates the connection with himself and with the world around.

Anything that supports the communication process, including medication, also furthers the change processes in the patient and thereby ensures a lasting recovery.

Cognitive-Behavioral Therapy (CBT)

CBT has been shown to be effective when used alone or in combination with medication. Patients receiving CBT work collaboratively with their therapists to learn specific skills to solve their problems and manage their emotions. In one recent study (1), patients were randomly assigned to treatment with either antidepressant medications alone or antidepressants combined with CBT. The recovery rates for patients who received combination therapy were better than for those who received medication alone (72.6% vs 62.5%), and this difference was particularly pronounced for patients who had severe and recurrent depressions (81% vs. 51%). Patients receiving combination treatment also had fewer serious side effects.

Psychodynamic Psychotherapy

Many patients with depression, anxiety disorders, and other psychiatric disorders are treated with combinations of psychodynamic psychotherapy and medication. Whether this is better than monotherapy is an empirical question that requires much more extensive research than is currently available.

Psychodynamic theorists and practitioners argued for some time that psychopharmacology offered only a superficial approach to treatment, a view which is no longer shared by the clear majority of psychodynamic psychotherapists. The few studies that have been done suggest that the combination of psychodynamic psychotherapy and medication may be superior for the treatment of mood and anxiety disorders, but most of these studies have small sample sizes and involve only short-term psychotherapy. (2)

References

1. Steven D. Hollon, Robert J. DeRubeis, Jan Fawcett, Jay D. Amsterdam, Richard C. Shelton, John Zajecka, Paula R. Young, Robert Gallop. Effect of Cognitive Therapy With Antidepressant Medications vs Antidepressants Alone on the Rate of Recovery in Major Depressive Disorder. JAMA Psychiatry, 2014; 71 (10): 1157.

2. Gorman JM. Combining Psychodynamic Psychotherapy and Pharmacotherapy. Psychodynamic Psychiatry 2016 44, 2, 183-209.

Suicide Prevention

Good communication can prevent suicide. This applies to the interaction between doctor and patient, but also how patients communicate with themselves and their environment. Public awareness about the risks of suicide can be helpful in enabling people to notice a problem early. Suicide is the third leading cause of death in youth and more than 90% of suicides in depressed youth are untreated at the time of death. [23]

Suicide usually requires the presence of a psychiatric condition. If an individual is in a good place emotionally and there are no other psychiatric conditions, suicide generally does not occur. But there is often an additional constellation of factors which lays the foundation for such a desperate act. One such factor is a disconnect from the outside world. A loss of connectedness means a loss of exchange of meaningful messages, which reduces the amount of meaning one experiences. Meaningful messages contain information that has the potential to bring about a change in the state, thoughts or emotions of a recipient. All organisms, humans included, need this exchange to adapt and feel connected with their environment, internally and externally. An important suicide prevention is thus to help the individual to better connect with oneself and with the world around.

Suicide and Mental Health

The important element for public awareness is that there is a solid link between mental illness and suicide. They cannot really be seen separately. People who have suicidal thoughts and the intention to act on them usually suffer from a mental health condition. Unfortunately, this is often overlooked. Depressions, psychoses, dissociative conditions and more often remain untreated, either because the patient does not seek treatment, or a correct diagnosis is never made. Besides raising public awareness for mental health, it is important to educate patients on the opportunities of treatment and the individual benefits this can offer.

Depression can lead to the low mood and emotional disconnectedness which can increase the pain and pressure to have suicidal thoughts. However, often it also leads to a reduction in energy and the initiative to act, which could reduce the risk of actually going through with a suicidal idea. This is why there has been a discussion for many years whether giving antidepressants, which can raise the activity level before raising the mood, could increase the risk of suicide in more severely depressed patients. Most clinicians would now say that it is usually better to give an antidepressant, but that one may need to do this under supervision or in a hospital in certain cases. Better communication not only works here against the depression but can also lower the risk of suicidal thoughts and actions. Sometimes just talking about the suffering and pain from the depression can be helpful for the patient, as long as the patient feels that this brings about a change, rather than just going in circles. For several communication techniques in practice the reader is referred to the author's books on psychotherapeutic technique and communication-focused therapy (CFT) of the same titles.

Various forms of psychosis can make the world a scary and possibly unbearable place because own negative thoughts and emotions can seem real. Fearful thoughts, for example, can turn into the conviction that one is being pursued in real life. Here communication plays a significant role again. A psychotic patient has lost, either partially or fully, the capacity to reflect on the own internal communication and to identify the sources of information, whether sensory, perceptual, emotional or thoughts, which can lead to the situation just mentioned. Practicing communication between patient and therapist and reflecting on it can help the patient to adjust also the internal communication. However, a meaningful interaction by itself, can give the patient a greater emotional safety and also a greater sense of efficacy in the shared reality by communicating about own needs, wants, emotions, aspirations, and so on. It is just important not to overwhelm a patient suffering from psychosis, who may have less solid boundaries between the shared reality and the inner worlds.

Prevention

Depression and other psychiatric disorders are underrecognized and undertreated in the primary care setting. (1,2) This is a significant problem because most suicides have had contact with a primary care physician within a month of death. (3,4) An Australian program that trained primary care physicians to recognize and respond to psychological distress and suicidal ideation in young people increased identification of suicidal patients by 130% (determined by the Depressive Symptom Inventory– Suicidality Subscale score), without changes in treatment or management strategies. (5)

Communication

Communication is important in preventing suicide. It helps to identify people who may be at risk of committing suicide, to establish a therapeutic and supportive relationship with them, and to give them the sense that they are understood and not alone and hope. However, as already mentioned, communication plays a much larger role as well. Communication is how we can notice and see meaning in things, including interpersonal relationships. Information is important because it helps one to adapt to and shape new situations. Meaningful can help take away the sense of loneliness and give a greater sense of connectedness with life. The last point is particularly important in preventing suicides in the relatively young (late adolescence, early adulthood) and relatively old (retirees, widows and widowers). Generally, if there is a change in life, effective communication with oneself and others can help to bridge the transition into new circumstances.

Screening

Screening aims to identify at-risk individuals and direct them to treatment. Often it is helpful to screen for suicide risk when screening for mental health conditions that are typically correlated with a higher risk of suicide, such as depression. Screening in localized geographic areas results in more treatment of depression and lower suicide rates. (8-10)

Administering instruments for depression, suicidal ideation, or suicidal acts to high school students and other youth groups is reported to double the number of known at-risk individuals. (6) The US Preventive Services Task Force (USPSTF) review of studies of depression screening in adults in primary health care settings found a 10% to 47% increase in rates of detection and diagnosis of depression with the use of screening tools. There is no evidence that screening youth for suicide induces suicidal thinking or behavior. (7)

Pharmacotherapy

Psychiatric disorders are present in at least 90% of suicides and more than 80% are untreated at time of death. (11,12) Treating mood and other psychiatric disorders is a central component of suicide prevention. Higher prescription rates of antidepressants correlate with decreasing suicide rates in adults or youth in Hungary, (13) Sweden, (14) Australia, (15) and the United States. (16,17)

Antidepressants

Antidepressants save Lives

Geographic regions or demographic groups with the highest selective serotonin reuptake inhibitor prescription rates have the lowest suicide rates in the United States (18) and Australia. (19) Suicide rates in 27 countries fell most markedly in countries that had the greatest increase min selective serotonin reuptake inhibitor prescriptions. (20) Patient population studies report lower suicide attempt rates in adults treated with antidepressant medication [21] and in adolescents after 6 months of antidepressant treatment compared with less than two months of treatment. [22]

Antipsychotics

Antipsychotics can be important to help a patient to experience the shared reality more clearly, which also makes it easier to act and interact in the world. While some of their side effects can lower the experience of emotional connectedness with oneself (45) and possibly even interfere with the communication with others in some areas, on balance they can help a patient suffering from psychotic symptoms to be more mentally more present in the shared reality, which improves also the interactions with others.

Psychotherapy

Promising results in reducing repetition of suicidal behavior and improving treatment adherence exist for cognitive therapy, (24) problem-solving therapy, (25) intensive care plus outreach, (26) and interpersonal psychotherapy, (27) compared with standard aftercare.

Psychotherapy alone or in combination with some antidepressants can be an effective treatment for depression, for suicidal ideation, for suicide attempts in borderline personality disorder, and for preventing new attempts after a suicide attempt. More needs to be known about the combinations of psychotherapeutic and pharmacologic interventions for short-and long-term outcomes for suicidal patients.

After a suicide attempt, better structured collaboration between hospitals and teams providing follow-up care may improve compliance with treatment and decrease new attempts, but essential elements of post-suicide attempt interventions are yet to be identified.

Cognitive Therapy

Cognitive therapy halved the reattempt rate in suicide attempters compared with those receiving usual care. (28) In borderline personality disorder, dialectical behavioral therapy (29) and psychoanalytically oriented partial hospitalization (30) improved treatment adherence and reduced suicidal behavior compared with standard after care.

Intermediate outcomes such as hopelessness and depressive symptoms improve with problem solving therapy, and suicidal ideation is decreased with interpersonal psychotherapy, cognitive behavior therapy, and dialectical behavioral therapy. (31)

Communication-Focused Therapy (CFT)

Communication-Focused Therapy (CFT) has been developed by the author to focus more closely on the mechanism which is the engine of change in many flavors of psychotherapy, from cognitive behavioral therapy (CBT) to psychodynamic psychotherapy (36). Although psychotherapy started as the 'talking cure' progressively less attention has been paid to the process of exchanging messages. While psychodynamic psychotherapy developed several concepts relying on communication mechanisms, such as transference and counter-transference, and also delineated some possible internal communication processes, later therapeutic schools, including cognitive, behavioral and interpersonal therapy, focused less on the fundamental process of the exchange of messages to bring about change. CFT tries to correct this. CFT has been described by the author for various mental health conditions (37).

Focusing one the communication process seems to be particularly helpful in suicidal patients, because the connectedness itself, if it is meaningful to the patient, probably has anti-suicidal properties. It is unfortunate that in many hospitals there are elaborate programs trying to implement specific therapeutic models, rather than focusing on the general process, which helps directly, and is the one which by necessity underlies any successful therapeutic process. Communication can be quite complex and takes considerable experience to understand. However, at the same time anyone has the tools to use it, and it would probably help to reduce suicides if it were used more, especially in larger healthcare centers which quite often are perceived as rather anonymous and interaction averse.

Follow-Up Care

Many psychiatric disorders, including depression, are chronic and recurrent and compliance with maintenance medication is often poor. Reduction of the number of psychiatric inpatient beds in Norway as part of a program of deinstitutionalization of psychiatric inpatients resulted in an increased suicide rate in the year after discharge with a standardized mortality ratio of 133 (95% confidence interval, 90.1-190.7) in men and 208.5 (95% confidence interval, 121.5-333.9) in women. (32)

Other interventions for those who attempt suicide, including telephone follow-up, intensive psychosocial follow-up, and video education plus family therapy, resulted in no difference between standard aftercare and intervention groups in rate of reattempt or reemergent suicidal ideation. (33-35)

References

1. Hirschfeld RMA, Keller M, Panico S, et al. The National Depressive and Manic-Depressive Association consensus statement on the undertreatment of depression. JAMA. 1997;277:333-340.

2. Goldman LS, Nielsen NH, Champion HC. Awareness, diagnosis, and treatment of depression. J Gen Intern Med. 1999;14:569-580.

3. Luoma JB, Martin CE, Pearson JL. Contact with mental health and primary care providers before suicide: a review of the evidence. Am J Psychiatry. 2002; 159:909-916.

4. Andersen UA, Andersen M, Rosholm JU, Gram LF. Contacts to the health care system prior to suicide: a comprehensive analysis using registers for general and psychiatric hospital admissions, contacts to general practitioners and practicing specialists and drug prescriptions. Acta Psychiatr Scand. 2000;102: 126-134.

5. Pfaff JJ, Acres JG, McKelvey RS. Training general practitioners to recognise and respond to psychological distress and suicidal ideation in young people. Med J Aust. 2001;174:222-226.

7. Gould MS, Marrocco FA, Kleinman M, et al. Evaluating iatrogenic risk of youth suicide screening programs: a randomized controlled trial. JAMA. 2005; 293:1635-1643.

8. Oyama H, Koida J, Sakashita T, Kudo K. Community-based prevention for suicide in elderly by depression screening and follow-up. Community Ment Health J. 2004;40:249-263.

10. Rutz W, Von Knorring L, Wálinder J. Frequency of suicide on Gotland after systematic postgraduate education of general practitioners. Acta Psychiatr Scand. 1989;80:151-154.

11. Henriksson S, Boethius G, Isacsson G. Suicides are seldom prescribed antidepressants: findings from a prospective prescription database in Jamtland county, Sweden, 1985-95. Acta Psychiatr Scand. 2001;103: 301-306.

12. Lonnqvist JK, Henriksson MM, Isometsa ET, et al. Mental disorders and suicide prevention. Psychiatry Clin Neurosci. 1995;49(suppl 1):S111-S116.

13. Rihmer Z, Belso N, Kalmar S. Antidepressants and suicide prevention in Hungary. Acta Psychiatr Scand. 2001;103:238-239.

14. Carlsten A, Waern M, Ekedahl A, Ranstam J. Antidepressant medication and suicide in Sweden. Pharmacoepidemiol Drug Saf. 2001;10:525-530.

15. Hall WD, Mant A, Mitchell PB, Rendle VA, Hickie IB, McManus P. Association between antidepressant prescribing and suicide in Australia, 1991-2000: trend analysis. BMJ. 2003;326:1008.

16. Gibbons RD, Hur K, Bhaumik DK, Mann JJ. The relationship between antidepressant medication use and rate of suicide. Arch Gen Psychiatry. 2005;65:165- 172.

17. Olfson M, Shaffer D, Marcus SC, Greenberg T. Relationship between antidepressant medication treatment and suicide in adolescents. Arch Gen Psychiatry. 2003;60:978-982.

18. Gibbons RD, Hur K, Bhaumik DK, Mann JJ. The relationship between antidepressant medication use and rate of suicide. Arch Gen Psychiatry. 2005;65:165- 172.

19. Hall WD, Mant A, Mitchell PB, Rendle VA, Hickie IB, McManus P. Association between antidepressant prescribing and suicide in Australia, 1991-2000: trend analysis. BMJ. 2003;326:1008.

20. Ludwig J, Marcotte DE. Anti-depressants, suicide, and drug regulation.J Policy Anal Manage. 2005; 24:249-272.

21. Simon GE, Savarino J, Operskalski B, Wang PS. Suicide risk during antidepressant treatment. Am J Psychiatry. In press.

22. Valuck RJ, Libby AM, Sills MR, Giese AA, Allen RR. Antidepressant treatment and risk of suicide attempt by adolescents with major depressive disorder: a propensity-adjusted retrospective cohort study. CNS Drugs. 2004;18:1119-1132.

23. Leon AC, Marzuk PM, Tardiff K, Teres JJ. Paroxetine, other antidepressants, and youth suicide in New York City: 1993 through 1998.J Clin Psychiatry. 2004;65:915-918.

24. Brown GK, Ten Have TR, Henriques GR, et al. Cognitive therapy for the prevention of suicide attempts: a randomized controlled trial. JAMA. 2005;294:563- 570.

25. Hawton K, Townsend E, Arensman E, et al. Psychosocial versus pharmacological treatments for deliberate self harm. Cochrane Database Syst Rev. 2002: CD001764.

26. Hawton K, Townsend E, Arensman E, et al. Psychosocial versus pharmacological treatments for deliberate self harm. Cochrane Database Syst Rev. 2002: CD001764.

27. Guthrie E, Kapur N, Mackway-Jones K, et al. Randomised controlled trial of brief psychological intervention after deliberate self poisoning. BMJ. 2001;323: 135-138.

28. Brown GK, Ten Have TR, Henriques GR, et al. Cognitive therapy for the prevention of suicide attempts: a randomized controlled trial. JAMA. 2005;294:563- 570.

30. Bateman A, Fonagy P. Treatment of borderline personality disorder with psychoanalytically oriented partial hospitalization: an 18-month follow-up. Am J Psychiatry. 2001;158:36-42.

32. Hansen V, Jacobsen BK, Arnesen E. Cause-specific mortalityinpsychiatricpatients after deinstitutionalisation. Br J Psychiatry. 2001;179:438-443.

33. Cedereke M, Monti K, Ojehagen A. Telephone contact with patients in the year after a suicide attempt: does it affect treatment attendance and outcome? a randomised controlled study. Eur Psychiatry. 2002;17:82-91.

34. Allard R, Marshall M, Plante MC. Intensive follow-up does not decrease the risk of repeat suicide attempts. Suicide Life Threat Behav. 1992;22:303-314.

35. Rotheram-Borus MJ, Piacentini J, Cantwell C, Belin TR, Song J. The 18-month impact of an emergency room intervention for adolescent female suicide attempters. J Consult Clin Psychol. 2000;68: 1081-1093.

36. Haverkampf CJ CBT and Psychodynamic Psychotherapy - A Comparison. J Psychiatry Psychotherapy Communication 2017 Sept 30 6(2)61-68

37. Haverkampf CJ. Communication-Focused Therapy (CFT). 2nd ed. London: Psychiatry Psychotherapy Communication Publishing Ltd; 2017.

Monitoring for Antidepressants

All Antidepressants

General Physical Assessment

blood pressure, heart rate, height, weight, BMI at least every 6 months

> Venlafaxine has been associated with elevated blood pressure, especially at high doses (300-375mg/day).

> In one study, the rates for 'postural hypotension' were as follows: Nefazodone (2.8%), tricyclic antidepressants (10.9%), SSRI (1.1%), and placebo (0.8%). (1)

temperature and respiratory rate as clinically indicated

Pregnancy Status

in females of childbearing age ask for reproductive status including last menstrual period, last pelvic exam/pap smear and contraceptive use

Renal function testing

medications excreted renally include

> bupropion
> duloxetine/Cymbalta(R)
> venlafaxine
> mirtazapine
> tricyclic antidepressants
> escitalopram

and others

Liver enzymes (Aminotransferases)

Although an infrequent event, drug-induced liver injury (DILI) from antidepressant drugs may be irreversible. Aminotransferase surveillance is the most useful tool for detecting DILI, and prompt discontinuation of the drug responsible is essential. (2)

The antidepressants associated with greater risks of hepatotoxicity are iproniazid, nefazodone, phenelzine, imipramine, amitriptyline, duloxetine, bupropion, trazodone, tianeptine, and agomelatine. The antidepressants that seem to have the least potential for hepatotoxicity are citalopram, escitalopram, paroxetine, and fluvoxamine. Cross-toxicity has been described, mainly for tricyclic and tetracyclic antidepressants. (2)

Serotonin Syndrome

Assess for the risk of the potentially lethal serotonin syndrome. The symptoms include abdominal pain, diarrhoea, flushing, sweating, hyperthermia, lethargy, mental status changes, tremor, renal failure, shock

Be cautious when combining serotonergic medications such as triptans for migraines e.g. Imitrex, synthetic opioids (tramadol/Ultram®, methadone), the antibiotic linezolid/Zyvox®

Other common side effects

Other potential side effects that may require action and should be specifically asked for

> changes in appetite
> sleep disturbances
> sexual function (menstrual disturbances, libido disturbances or erectile/ejaculatory disturbances)
> orthostatic hypotension

Weight Gain

Abdominal girth should be measured at least every 6 months, particularly with the TCAs including

> amitriptyline
> clomipramine
> doxepin
> imipramine

and mirtazapine.

Bone Density

Depression and some treatments including SSRIs have been linked to a decrease in bone density. If indicated, refer for bone density monitoring and treatment to reduce bone loss (e.g. calcium, vitamin D, weight bearing exercise, etc.)

Past Medical History

Review Past Medical History Including Review of All Medications at least annually

- assess allergies, current medications including over-the-counter and herbal supplements
- surgeries, hospitalizations

Selective Serotonin Reuptake Inhibitors (SSRIs)

e.g. citalopram, escitalopram, fluoxetine, fluvoxamine, sertraline

Bleeding Risk

- Identify whether concomitant medications may affect clotting.
- SSRIs may potentiate the hypoprothrombinemic effects by inhibiting serotonin uptake by platelets.
- Monitor for signs of bleeding.

Fasting Blood Glucose

Use of SSRIs was associated with lower insulin secretion in nondiabetic participants and an increased risk of insulin dependence in type 2 diabetics in older adults. However, additional studies are required to confirm our results. (4)

QT Interval

ECG if indicated.

SSRIs may in combination with some medication lead to QT interval prolongation.

Tricyclic antidepressants (TCAs)

e.g. amitriptyline, desipramine, imipramine, nortriptyline, protriptyline

Electrocardiogram (ECG)

- TCAs can cause arrhythmias, and heart block in patients with pre-existing conduction disorders.
- Evaluate patients for cardiac risk factors such as a personal history of heart disease or syncope, a family history of sudden death under the age of 40, or congenital long QT syndrome. Avoid TCAs if recent MI, history of ventricular arrhythmia or other conduction defects.
- Baseline ECG if cardiac risk factors are present or patient is older than 50 and a follow up ECG if the patient has symptoms associated with QT interval prolongation such as syncope

Drug plasma levels

drug interactions that can greatly elevate plasma levels

Thyroid

Thyroid Function at least annually

Tricyclic antidepressant drugs complex with iodine and thyroid peroxidase and deactivate them, induce deiodinase activity and interfere with the hypothalamo-pituitary-thyroid (HPT) axis by decreasing TSH response to TRH. (3)

Liver Function Tests

Fasting Blood Glucose

Lipid Panel

total cholesterol, LDL, triglycerides and HDL at baseline and as clinically indicated

The unfavorable effect of weight gain promoting antidepressants (e.g., tricyclics, mirtazapine) on serum lipid parameters (i.e., triglycerides and low-density lipoprotein cholesterol) is a consistent finding. Weight-neutral antidepressants (e.g., bupropion, venlafaxine, duloxetine), however, are less likely to disrupt the lipid milieu. (4)

Mirtazapine

Lipid Panel

- total cholesterol, LDL, triglycerides and HDL at baseline and as clinically indicated
- Mirtazapine is extensively metabolized in the liver. (5)

Fasting Blood Glucose

Weight

The antidepressant therapy with mirtazapine seems to be associated with a significant increase in body weight, body fat mass, and leptin concentration. In contrast to other psychotropic medications inducing weight gain, such as some second-generation antipsychotics, mirtazapine treatment is unlikely to influence the glucose homeostasis. (6)

(The risk of QT/QTc prolongation with the majority of newer non-SSRI antidepressants at therapeutic doses seems low. (6))

Serotonin Norepinephrine Reuptake Inhibitors (SNRIs)

e.g. Venlafaxine (Efexor®)

Blood Pressure

Venlafaxine has been associated with elevated blood pressure, especially at high doses (300-375mg/day). Although there are studies that cannot reproduce this observation. (7)

Norepinephrine Dopamine Reuptake Inhibitors

e.g. Bupropion

Screen for history of seizures

- Bupropion is known to reduce seizure thresholds, with a seizure rate of about 1 in 1000 subjects treated. (8)

- Bupropion is contraindicated if there is a pre-existing seizure disorder. It should be avoided in those at higher risk for seizures, including those undergoing abrupt discontinuation of alcohol or benzodiazepines/sedatives, those with eating disorders including anorexia or bulimia, head trauma or brain tumors.

Blood pressure

Assess blood pressure before initiating treatment with Wellbutrin XL, and monitor periodically during treatment (9)

MAO Inhibitors

e.g. phenelzine, tranylcypromine, moclobemide, selegiline

Hepatic function

at least the irreversible non-selective MAO inhibitors: phenelzine, tranylcypromine, etc

Renal function

at least the irreversible non-selective MAO inhibitors: phenelzine, tranylcypromine, etc

Assess diet

to avoid the tyramine reaction

(The selective monoamine oxidase-B inhibitor selegiline and the selective and reversible inhibitor of monoamine oxidase-A (RIMA) seem to have a much lower or no risk of causing a hypertensive crisis (10)

Avoid tyramine containing foods and caffeine during treatment and for 2 weeks after discontinuing

Combinations may cause severe headaches, increased blood pressure or irregular heartbeat. Tyramine-containing foods to avoid include aged cheeses, aged/processed meats and pickled fish, beer, ale, wine, sherry, hard liquor, liquors, avocados, bananas, figs, raisins, soy sauce, miso soup, yeast/protein extracts, bean curd, or over-ripe fruit. Also, avoid caffeine including tea, coffee, chocolate or cola.

St John's Wort

Preparations containing St John's Wort should be treated like any other antidepressant. It is also advisable to check the liver enzymes at larger intervals and proceed as in the section for "all antidepressants".

One needs to keep in mind the risk of phototoxicity when the skin is exposed to sunlight.

Other drugs may be metabolized differently, since St John's Wort contains substances that can be potent enzyme inducers. (11)

References

1. http://www.drugs.com/

2. Voican CS, Corruble E, Naveau S, Perlemuter G. Antidepressant-induced liver injury: a review for clinicians. American Journal of Psychiatry. 2014 Apr;171(4):404-15.

3. Khalil RB, Richa S. Thyroid adverse effects of psychotropic drugs: a review. Clinical neuropharmacology. 2011 Nov 1;34(6):248-55.

4. McIntyre RS, Soczynska JK, Konarski JZ, Kennedy SH. The effect of antidepressants on lipid homeostasis: a cardiac safety concern? Expert opinion on drug safety. 2006 Jul 1;5(4):523-37.

5. Laimer M, Kramer-Reinstadler K, Rauchenzauner M, Lechner-Schoner T, Strauss R, Engl J, Deisenhammer EA, Hinterhuber H, Patsch JR, Ebenbichler CF. Effect of mirtazapine treatment on body composition and metabolism. The Journal of clinical psychiatry. 2006 Mar;67(3):421-4.

6. Anttila SA, Leinonen EV. A review of the pharmacological and clinical profile of mirtazapine. CNS drug reviews. 2001 Sep 1;7(3):249-64.

7. Mbaya P, Alam F, Ashim S, Bennett D. Cardiovascular effects of high dose venlafaxine XL in patients with major depressive disorder. Human Psychopharmacology: Clinical and Experimental. 2007 Apr 1;22(3):129-33.

8. Jasiak NM, Bostwick JR. Risk of QT/QTc prolongation among newer non-SSRI antidepressants. Annals of Pharmacotherapy. 2014 Dec 1;48(12):1620-8.

8. Wooltorton E. Bupropion (Zyban, Wellbutrin SR): reports of deaths, seizures, serum sickness. Canadian Medical Association Journal. 2002 Jan 8;166(1):68-.

9. http://www.fda.gov/Safety/MedWatch/SafetyInformation

10. Yamada M, Yasuhara H. Clinical pharmacology of MAO inhibitors: safety and future. Neurotoxicology. 2004 Jan 31;25(1):215-21.

11. Moore LB, Goodwin B, Jones SA, Wisely GB, Serabjit-Singh CJ, Willson TM, Collins JL, Kliewer SA. St. John's wort induces hepatic drug metabolism through activation of the pregnane X receptor. Proceedings of the National Academy of Sciences. 2000 Jun 20;97(13):7500-2.

Monitoring for Antipsychotics

All Atypical Antipsychotics

Because of the known metabolic side effects that occur in patients taking an atypical antipsychotic, baseline and periodic monitoring is recommended.

BMI and waist circumference

should be recorded at baseline and tracked throughout treatment. Ideally, obtain measurements

>   monthly for the first 3 months of therapy, or
>   after any medication adjustments, then
>   at 6 months, and
>   annually thereafter.

Encourage patients to track their own weight.

HbA1c and fasting plasma glucose levels

should be measured at baseline and throughout the course of treatment. Obtain another set of measurements at 3 months, then annually thereafter, unless the patient develops type 2 diabetes mellitus.

Lipid Panel

Obtaining a lipid panel at baseline and periodically throughout the course of treatment is recommended. After baseline measurement, another panel should be taken

- at 3 months and
- annually thereafter.

Guidelines of the American Diabetes Association recommend a fasting lipid panel every 5 year—however, good clinical practice dictates obtaining a lipid panel annually.

ECG Monitoring

Mellaril (thioridazine), Serentil (mesoridazine) and Orap (pimozide) should not be prescribed for anyone with known heart disease.

Geodon can be prescribed in patients with heart disease, but you should get a baseline ECG, and get follow-up ECG. In patients with no cardiac history, no screening ECG is required.

Prolactin

Patients on Risperdal and most first-generation antipsychotics should be asked screening questions about symptoms of elevated prolactin. For women, ask about changes in menstruation or libido, and whether they have noticed a milk discharge from breasts. For men, ask about libido and sexual dysfunction. Order prolactin levels only if screening questions indicate possible hyperprolactinemia.

Neuroleptic Malignant Syndrome (NMS)

NMS is usually caused by antipsychotic drug use, and a wide range of drugs can result in NMS. Individuals using butyrophenones (such as haloperidol and droperidol) or phenothiazines (such as promethazine and chlorpromazine) are reported to be at greatest risk. However, various atypical antipsychotics such as clozapine, olanzapine, risperidone, quetiapine, and ziprasidone have also been implicated in cases. NMS is associated with elevated creatinine phosphokinase (CPK) levels. (2)

The first symptoms of neuroleptic malignant syndrome are usually muscle cramps and tremors, fever, symptoms of autonomic nervous system instability such as unstable blood pressure, and sudden changes in mental status (agitation, delirium, or coma). Once symptoms appear, they may progress rapidly and reach peak intensity in as little as three days. These symptoms can last anywhere from eight hours to forty days. The muscular symptoms are most likely caused by blockade of the dopamine receptor D2, leading to abnormal function of the basal ganglia similar to that seen in Parkinson's disease.

Symptoms are sometimes misinterpreted by doctors as symptoms of mental illness which can result in delayed treatment. NMS is less likely if a person has previously been stable for a period of time on antipsychotics, especially in situations where the dose has not been changed and there are no issues of noncompliance or consumption of psychoactive substances known to worsen psychosis.

- Increased body temperature >38 °C (>100.4 °F), or
- Confused or altered consciousness
- Diaphoresis

- Rigid muscles
- Autonomic imbalance

Aripiprazole

e.g. Abilify ®

Weight

Baseline, 6 months, then yearly

Glucose

Baseline glucose (fasting not necessary); then yearly

Lipids

Baseline fasting lipid panel every 2 years.

CPK

if indicated

Neuroleptic malignant syndrome is typically characterized by high fever, muscular rigidity, and mental status changes, along with characteristic laboratory findings including creatinine phosphokinase (CPK) elevation and often leukocytosis.

Olanzapine

e.g. Zyprexa ®

Weight

Determine BMI (body mass index, defined as weight divided by height) at baseline, once a month for the first three months, then every three months

Glucose

1. Baseline fasting glucose (below 100 is normal, 100-125 is pre-diabetes, above 126 is diabetes). If your patient can't manage to get to the lab before eating, order an HbA1c, which is a measure of long term glucose control.
2. Follow-up fasting glucose 4 months after starting med and then yearly, unless patients are gaining weight: if so, continue Q 4 mo. monitoring.

Ask patients about polyuria or polydipsia to monitor for diabetes.

Lipids

Baseline fasting lipid panel: total cholesterol, low-density lipoprotein (LDL) and HDL cholesterol, and triglyceride levels. Check lipids again 3 months later, then every 2 years; refer to PCP if LDL is higher than 130 mg/dl.

CPK

if indicated

Neuroleptic malignant syndrome is typically characterized by high fever, muscular rigidity, and mental status changes, along with characteristic laboratory findings including creatinine phosphokinase (CPK) elevation and often leukocytosis.

Quetiapine

e.g. Seroquel ®

Weight

Determine BMI (body mass index, defined as weight divided by height) at baseline, once a month for the first three months, then every three months.

Glucose

1. Baseline fasting glucose (below 100 is normal, 100-125 is pre-diabetes, above 126 is diabetes). If your patient can't manage to get to the lab before eating, order an HbA1c, which is a measure of long term glucose control.
2. Follow-up fasting glucose 4 months after starting med and then yearly, unless patients are gaining weight: if so, continue Q 4 mo. monitoring.

Ask patients about polyuria or polydipsia to monitor for diabetes.

Lipids

Baseline fasting lipid panel: total cholesterol, low-density lipoprotein (LDL) and HDL cholesterol, and triglyceride levels. Check lipids again 3 months later, then every 2 years; refer to PCP if LDL is higher than 130 mg/dl.

CPK

if indicated

Neuroleptic malignant syndrome is typically characterized by high fever, muscular rigidity, and mental status changes, along with characteristic laboratory findings including creatinine phosphokinase (CPK) elevation and often leukocytosis.

Risperidone

e.g Risperdal ®

Weight

Determine BMI (body mass index, defined as weight divided by height) at baseline, once a month for the first three months, then every three months

Glucose

1. Baseline fasting glucose (below 100 is normal, 100-125 is pre-diabetes, above 126 is diabetes). If your patient can't manage to get to the lab before eating, order an HbA1c, which is a measure of long term glucose control.
2. Follow-up fasting glucose 4 months after starting med and then yearly, unless patients are gaining weight: if so, continue Q 4 mo. monitoring.

Ask patients about polyuria or polydipsia to monitor for diabetes.

Lipids

Baseline fasting lipid panel: total cholesterol, low-density lipoprotein (LDL) and HDL cholesterol, and triglyceride levels. Check lipids again 3 months later, then every 2 years; refer to PCP if LDL is higher than 130 mg/dl.

CPK

if indicated

Neuroleptic malignant syndrome is typically characterized by high fever, muscular rigidity, and mental status changes, along with characteristic laboratory findings including creatinine phosphokinase (CPK) elevation and often leukocytosis.

Paliperidone

e.g. Invega ®

Weight

Determine BMI (body mass index, defined as weight divided by height) at baseline, once a month for the first three months, then every three months

Glucose

1. Baseline fasting glucose (below 100 is normal, 100-125 is pre-diabetes, above 126 is diabetes). If your patient can't manage to get to the lab before eating, order an HbA1c, which is a measure of long term glucose control

2. Follow-up fasting glucose 4 months after starting med and then yearly, unless patients are gaining weight: if so, continue Q 4 mo. monitoring.

Ask patients about polyuria or polydipsia to monitor for diabetes.

Lipids

Baseline fasting lipid panel: total cholesterol, low-density lipoprotein (LDL) and HDL cholesterol, and triglyceride levels. Check lipids again 3 months later, then every 2 years; refer to PCP if LDL is higher than 130 mg/dl.

CPK

if indicated

Neuroleptic malignant syndrome is typically characterized by high fever, muscular rigidity, and mental status changes, along with characteristic laboratory findings including creatinine phosphokinase (CPK) elevation and often leukocytosis.

Ziprasidone

Weight

Baseline, 6 months, then yearly

Glucose

Baseline glucose (fasting not necessary); then yearly

Lipids

Baseline fasting lipid panel every 2 years

CPK

if indicated

Neuroleptic malignant syndrome is typically characterized by high fever, muscular rigidity, and mental status changes, along with characteristic laboratory findings including creatinine phosphokinase (CPK) elevation and often leukocytosis.

References

1. Zeier K, Connell R, Resch W, Thomas CJ. Recommendations for lab monitoring of atypical antipsychotics. Current Psychiatry. 2013 Sep 1;12(9):51.

2. Strawn JR, Keck Jr, MD PE, Caroff SN. Neuroleptic malignant syndrome. American Journal of Psychiatry. 2007 Jun;164(6):870-6.

www.ingramcontent.com/pod-product-compliance
Lightning Source LLC
Chambersburg PA
CBHW071425180526
45170CB00001B/231